Advance praise for
CRACKED OPEN
Liberty, Fertility, and the Pursuit of High Tech Babies

"*Cracked Open* is a provocative look at what happens when feminism's promise of choice collides with the limitations of reproductive science. Miriam Zoll was confident that she could postpone pregnancy to pursue her career. But once she was ready to start a family she discovered that, despite technological advances and positive cultural support for 'older motherhood,' fertility clinics couldn't deliver the miracle she was counting on. Her story is a powerful reminder that as long as biology can trump personal aspirations, American women, even in the 21st century, cannot fully control their lives."
—**Letty Cottin Pogrebin, co-founder,** *Ms. Magazine*; **co-founder, National Women's Political Caucus; author of** *How to be a Friend to a Friend Who's Sick*

"*Cracked Open* tells the whole truth about the brave new world of ART (Assisted Reproductive Technologies)—and this truth isn't nearly as rosy as we've all been led to believe. I highly recommend this book to everyone truly concerned about the hearts and souls of humanity."
—**Christiane Northrup, M.D., Ob/Gyn physician;** *New York Times* **bestselling author of** *Women's Bodies, Women's Wisdom* **and** *The Wisdom of Menopause*

"Creating a baby has gone from one of the most intimate acts and private decisions women make to a high tech industry involving dozens of actors with personal and public consequences rarely revealed. In a skillful melding of personal story and medical and policy facts, Miriam Zoll asks all the right questions about the ethics of assisted reproductive technology and the place baby making has in women's lives and identity."
—**Frances Kissling, president, Center for Health, Ethics and Social Policy; former president, Catholics for Choice**

"*Cracked Open* is a compelling narrative that speaks for a generation of women who, like the author, delayed parenthood only to find themselves

immersed in the over-hyped world of America's 'Wild West' of reproductive medicine. Miriam Zoll convincingly indicts many current
practices in the IVF and egg donation industry, making her book a must
read both for anyone contemplating fertility treatments, and for those
who believe that reproductive medicine is badly in need of reform."
—George J. Annas, professor of health law, bioethics & human rights,
Boston University; author of *The Rights of Patients*

"*Cracked Open* is both a touching love story and a riveting account of one
couple's heartbreaking encounters with the virtually unregulated, non-
transparent and profit-driven world of reproductive medicine. Although
the failures of assisted reproductive technology are far more common
than the successes, first-person accounts of the often-devastating
consequences of entering this high-tech world remain all too rare. But
finally, here is a writer with the courage to reveal the intensely personal
drama of confronting infertility and medicine's inflated promises. The
reader's heart will be 'cracked open,' as were Zoll's and her husband's, as
they learned what it means to be 'real' parents. This memoir is a powerful
21st century saga that should serve as the catalyst for a long-overdue critical public dialogue on the health risks and social costs of the emergence
of an industry based on creating human life for profit."
—Diane Beeson, PhD, Alliance for Humane Biotechnology, professor
emerita, Department of Sociology, California State University, East Bay

"Miriam Zoll's book, *Cracked Open*, is a powerful, personal narrative
that details the hidden side of reproductive technologies in the United
States—a country that, for the most part, steadfastly refuses to regulate
its fertility industry, and thereby fails to protect the interests of women
and men who use assisted reproductive technologies, and the children
who are born from them."
—Françoise Baylis, professor and Canada research chair in bioethics and
philosophy, Dalhousie University; former member of the board of direc-
tors, Assisted Human Reproduction Canada, a federal oversight authority

"Heart wrenching, raw and honest—Miriam Zoll's thought-provoking
memoir brings us onto the emotional frontlines of life in the fast lane
of unregulated reproductive medicine in the United States. *Cracked*

Open powerfully illustrates the need for more public debate on the ethics, as well as the psychological and medical safety issues, related to donors, donor-conceived children and their parents. It is time that the fertility industry stopped focusing solely on achieving pregnancy and more on helping families in the most ethical and safe manner possible."
—**Wendy Kramer, co-founder and director, Donor Sibling Registry; co-author of** *Finding Our Families: A-First-of-its-Kind-Book for Donor-Conceived People and Their Families*

"Miriam Zoll's insightful memoir strikes at the heart of American women's desires and choices, and their quest to find wholeness through work, motherhood or a balance of both. *Cracked Open* is another sobering reminder that for couples hoping to create a biological family, trying sooner rather than later is the healthier option. With honesty and humility, the author offers her own story as proof that in order to get what we want, we sometimes have to learn to hear what we might not want to."
—**Amy Richards, co-founder, Third Wave Foundation; author of** *Opting In: Having a Child without Losing Yourself*

"The joy of becoming a parent through assisted reproduction is widely and warmly appreciated. But until now we've heard very little about those—the majority in all age groups—for whom high-tech fertility treatments fail. In *Cracked Open*, Miriam Zoll gives us an unblinking account of the emotional anguish, health complications, ethical quandaries and financial costs of her own journey into the fertility industry. *Cracked Open* is a wonderfully engaging memoir that also delivers vital insights into the consequences of our failure to adequately understand and regulate the business of assisted reproduction. It sits squarely in the powerful feminist tradition of revealing the political stakes of personal experience through sharing our most heartfelt stories."
—**Marcy Darnovsky, PhD, executive director, Center for Genetics and Society**

"*Cracked Open* takes an unvarnished look at the netherworld of assisted reproduction and its sometimes joyous outcomes but, more often, its attendant agonies, failures and resulting emotional traumas. Revealing a labyrinth of unverifiable hucksterism, unregulated therapies and

uninformed 'choices,' Miriam Zoll courageously reveals her own battles with anxiety, depression and post-traumatic stress disorder, and points the way for women in similar circumstances to heal themselves. This book can help couples make informed decisions and should be mandatory reading for both women and men entering their reproductive years."
—Alexander Sanger, Chair, International Planned Parenthood Council; former Goodwill Ambassador, United Nations Population Fund; Author, *Beyond Choice: Reproductive Freedom in the 21st Century*

"Unlike most traumas—which are single, horrific and devastating events—infertility is chronic, silent, and often hidden from the public eye. In her well-written, passionate, and funny memoir, Miriam Zoll shows us how this mournful health condition with its invasive medical treatments erodes one's sense of confidence and purpose, and eats away at relationships. *Cracked Open* is a must read for people coping with infertility—so they know they are not alone—and also for their friends and family, who often don't understand the true traumatic nature of what their loved ones are experiencing."
—Janet Jaffe, Ph.D., clinical psychologist, co-director, Center for Reproductive Psychology; co-author of *Reproductive Trauma* and *Unsung Lullabies: Understanding and Coping with Infertility*

"Finally, a book that speaks to the experience of the majority of reproductive health consumers who gamble their hearts and pocketbooks on fertility treatments but don't always win the jackpot they think they will. By telling her own story with honesty and humor, Miriam Zoll provides comfort, support—and warnings—to millions of women and men around the world coping with infertility."
—Naomi Cahn, the Harold H. Greene Professor of Law at George Washington University Law School; author of *Test Tube Families: Why the Fertility Market Needs Legal Regulation* and *The New Kinship: Constructing Donor-Conceived Families*

"Told in a refreshingly honest and forthcoming way, Miriam Zoll's eloquent account of the conflict between her desire for motherhood and the ethical issues around reproductive technologies could not have arrived at a better time. In *Cracked Open*, Zoll leads us behind the scenes

to slog through the personal and political ethics of creating human life in an unregulated marketplace, all the while dissecting through a critical lens how the reproductive industry markets its services to vulnerable women and men."
—**Rebecca Haimowitz amd Vaishali Sinha, co-directors/producers of the award-winning film** *Made in India*, **about the phenomenon of "outsourcing" surrogate mothers to India**

"Miriam Zoll has written a harrowing and moving account about her long ordeal in the maw of the unregulated U.S. infertility industry. *Cracked Open* is a love story set against a backdrop of the heartlessness of a cash-on-the-barrel-head medical trade that makes promises its technology infrequently keeps. Full of losses and spiritual insights, Zoll's book provides a sobering perspective not offered by brochures and baby-laden clinic websites. Anyone contemplating assisted reproduction owes it to themself to read *Cracked Open* first."
—**Gina Maranto, author** *Quest for Perfection: The Drive to Breed Better Human Beings*

"The world of assisted reproductive technologies is far more complex than it is often represented—spanning significant ethical, commercial, legal, human rights and cultural lines. *Cracked Open* takes us on an import personal journey through this world, one in which women and men are being offered many options but few explanations."
—**Jeremy Gruber, president, Council for Responsible Genetics**

"*Cracked Open* 'cracks open' the experimental process of IVF. Through a memoir about her own decision at the age of 40 to have children, Miriam Zoll unravels the brutal cultural effects and unfulfilled promises of the virtually unregulated IVF industry. Furthermore, her book rings a warning bell for those who expect that medical science will enable them to 'have it all.' As Zoll shows, we are no where near being able to make healthy babies on command, though in the process of trying, we are all too capable of messing with lives-to-be. Highly recommended."
—**S. Lochlain Jain, Associate Professor, Anthropology Department, Medical and Legal Anthropology, Stanford University; author,** *Injury: The Politics of Product Design and Safety Law in the United States*

CRACKED OPEN

Liberty, Fertility, and the Pursuit of High-Tech Babies

a memoir
by miriam zoll

Interlink Books

An imprint of Interlink Publishing Group, Inc.
Northampton, Massachusetts

First published in 2013 by

INTERLINK BOOKS
An imprint of Interlink Publishing Group, Inc.
46 Crosby Street, Northampton, Massachusetts 01060
www.interlinkbooks.com

Copyright © Miriam Zoll, 2013
Foreword copyright © Michele Goodwin and Judy Norsigian, 2013
Cover image copyright © Andrey Zametalov, Dreamstime.com (pregnant woman);
    Yanik Chauvin, Dreamstime.com (barcode)
Cover design: James McDonald, The Impress Group
Book design: Leyla Moushabeck

Library of Congress Cataloging-in-Publication Data
Zoll, Miriam.
 Cracked open : liberty, fertility, and the pursuit of high tech babies / by Miriam Zoll. -- First American edition.
    pages cm
Includes bibliographical references.
ISBN 978-1-56656-923-1
1. Human reproductive technology--History. 2. Reproductive technology--Popular works. 3. Infertility--Treatment--History. I. Title.
RG133.5.Z65 2013
618.1'7806--dc23

Printed and bound in the United States of America
10 9 8 7 6 5 4 3 2 1

To request a copy of our 48-page full-color catalog, please call 1-800-238-LINK, visit our website at www.interlinkbooks.com, email: info@interlinkbooks.com, or write to:
Interlink Publishing
46 Crosby Street
Northampton, MA 01060

*For M., whose open heart and acts
of love inspire me every day*

TABLE OF CONTENTS

FOREWORD

On September 5, 2012, a fifty-three-year-old grandmother from Chicago, Cindy Reutzel, birthed her daughter's baby—and said she would do it again. That same month reality television star Kim Kardashian announced that she was freezing her eggs for hopeful future use through a new technique unsupported by long-term women's and fetal health safety studies. A few days later, news circulated around the globe that the first mother-to-daughter womb transplants had been carried out in a hospital in Sweden. Some headlines touted the "miracle" that a woman might now have the ability to birth her own child from inside the same womb she herself was carried. The success of the procedure, doctors said, will not truly be "celebrated" unless the daughters actually birth babies from frozen embryo transplants at some point in the future.

ABC News called the womb transplant the "latest fertility feat" and raised questions about the ethics driving an industry that has grown into an ever-expanding multi-billion-dollar global business. Dr. James Goldfarb, director of University Hospital's Fertility Center in Cleveland, Ohio, and past president of the Society for Assisted Reproductive Technologies, was quoted as saying: "I've been around long enough to see some stuff we never imagined become sort of standard." Indeed, he is right, as even preteens with cancer participate in reproductive technology clinical trials to maximize their future ability to reproduce. Research teams in Chicago and Philadelphia are running clinical trials involving children as young as seven to develop and test the technology.[1]

Roll back to four years ago and news footage of "Octomom," an unemployed California mother of six who gave birth to octuplets. All fourteen of her children were born as a result of assisted reproductive technologies (ART) or in-vitro fertilization (IVF). As in prior cases of higher-order multiple births involving quintuplets and sextuplets, the nation rallied for this mysterious woman, who early on was anonymous. Soon after, the world came to know her: Nadya Suleman posed for the cameras and described how her fertility doctor had implanted not the "standard" one or two embryos into her womb (to reduce health risks) but six. As news about Suleman and her doctor's decision spread, unprecedented public debate erupted about the multiple ethical dilemmas surrounding the births. Kaiser Permanente's Bellflower Hospital, where the babies were born, deliberated about whether it should release the octuplets into the custody of a mother whose financial and psychological state was deemed perilous. The California Medical Board investigated the doctor, Michael Kamrava, and his Beverly Hills fertility clinic and eventually discovered that he had implanted not six but *twelve* embryos. Biomedical ethicists debated that, while Kamrava—whose license was revoked by the Board in July 2011—had acted with "gross negligence," he had not broken any laws. The truth is, there are hardly any laws now in place to break. The federal government requires only that clinics inform the Centers for Disease Control of their success rates.

In many respects it is ironic that while there have been so many recent attempts by policymakers to restrict women's access to legally protected contraception and abortion—two well-studied areas of reproductive health care—by comparison there are so few efforts underway to reign in misleading advertisements, conflicting fiduciary interests, and other conditions that surround the growing use of ARTs. Studies that have been conducted on higher-order multiple births have demonstrated increased risks for cerebral palsy, hearing and visual impairments, cognitive delays, and other traumas associated with crowded gestation. Some studies have even purported links to cancer for women who undergo aggressive "ovary blasting."

Cracked Open describes the ways in which the hyper-marketed, unregulated U.S. fertility industry has become popularly embedded in our lives and culture. Suleman's story—though bizarre and exaggerated—reveals a landscape of unmonitored medical practices and the absence of meaningful public dialogue as complex new technologies are introduced. This much-needed discourse would benefit the many Americans of reproductive age facing difficult challenges and profound decisions for themselves and their offspring. Walk into a room full of mostly urban professionals in their thirties and forties today and you're bound to find at least one couple—if not half a dozen—who have undergone fertility treatments or know someone who has. According to the U.S. National Survey of Family Growth, an estimated 7.3 million people experience infertility, or one out of every eight couples.[2] Data from the Centers for Disease Control suggest that 1.2 million women of reproductive age have had infertility-related medical appointments within the previous year, and an additional 10 percent had received infertility services at some time in their lives. Almost 12 percent of U.S. women aged 15 to 44 have reported using some type of infertility service.[3] The CDC's preliminary 2010 data show that nearly 150,000 ART cycles were reported at 443 clinics—about 91 percent of the total number of clinics in the United States. This resulted in an estimated 47,090 live births (delivery of one or more living infants) during that year.[4]

Thus, increasingly, Americans turn to ART usage—and for a variety of reasons. Many people desire to use the technologies responsibly and as a last resort at building a biologically linked family. Many more are simply desperate, while others are interested in convenience. Some couples that could otherwise produce offspring seek surrogates to avoid the morning sickness and physical changes brought on by pregnancies.

Regardless of the reasons, more and more Americans are swarming to the doorsteps of fertility clinics with their hopes high and their pockets bulging with cash. Many do not realize the extent to which they are participating in a vast experiment, where evidence-based medicine has yet to establish a reasonable foothold. They surrender their bodies, sexualities, and emotional lives to the doctors, syringes, and drugs that might lead them into parenthood. They sign up willingly because they believe—and the U.S. media reinforces their beliefs—that science and technology have finally outsmarted Mother Nature, and that concern for women's biological clocks is no longer relevant.

Cracked Open is a generational memoir that contextualizes coming of age at an extraordinary time in the United States—a time when birth control and abortion are still safe and legal, and women's participation in the world outside the home is the expected norm. Like Louise Brown, the world's first "test-tube baby," born in Britain in 1978, this generation became sexually active at the *same* time the media began to tout the wonders of IVF and related technologies. Now that these men and, in particular, women have entered the workforce, ART has reportedly advanced so much that many of them believe they can safely wait to have children until *after* a promotion at work, not before it. It is in

America, after all, where a fifty-six-year-old woman from Ohio birthed her triplet grandchildren and a woman from New Jersey birthed twins at the age of sixty. In America, it seems as if anything is possible.

But the truth is, despite the well-publicized success stories, many, if not most, fertility treatments do not result in live births, particularly for women over the age of forty. Through brutally honest storytelling, *Cracked Open* viscerally describes how fertility treatment failure and its accompanying emotional devastation are far more common than the covers of *People* magazine and many clinics would lead us to believe. While the "better" fertility centers now claim live birth rates of 50 percent or more, the national average remains about one-third. It is easy to misinterpret pregnancy rates—which are high but often end in miscarriage—as live birth rates, which are much lower in comparison. In August 2008, the U.S. Census reported that the number of women aged forty to forty-four who remain childless had doubled in a generation. In June 2006, 20 percent in that age group remained childless compared to only 10 percent thirty years earlier—prior to the increasing reliance of fertility treatments as a last resort.[5] The report does not cite specific reasons for the increase, but the growing trend among that age group to delay marriage and motherhood may be a factor. Today, more than 1 percent of all infants born in the U.S. each year are conceived using ART.

Globally, the industry is expanding through the fast-growing trend to hire financially disadvantaged women, especially in India, as gestational mothers or so-called "surrogate" mothers. As the birth mothers of the babies intended to be raised by other parents, these women are far from "surrogate"—their experiences of pregnancy and birth can't be called anything but "real" by any stretch of the imagination. India has already surpassed the United States as the world's "surrogacy capital," and about 25,000 couples from such countries as England and the United States now travel to India yearly for the less costly services provided by women who are often in desperate need of income. And on the demand side, although the media often refer to these trips overseas as "reproductive tourism," the journeys are anything but vacations for those who travel abroad and experience considerable stress and anxiety.

Cracked Open also draws important attention to the absence of adequate long-term safety data relevant to the health of children born from and women undergoing ART procedures like egg extraction, whether for themselves or others. A voluntary registry housed at Dartmouth Hitchcock Medical Center—the Infertility Family

Research Registry (www.ifrr-registry.org)—has for several years been seeking to increase data collection by tracking the health of a number of individuals engaged in ART treatments. Initially funded by the National Institutes of Health and now funded by the American Society for Reproductive Medicine (ASRM) and the Society for Assisted Reproductive Technology (SART), the Registry has yet to attract the participation of many young women responding to targeted egg donation ads on college campuses. If more fertility centers were to advertise the existence of the Registry as a way of encouraging participation, more volunteers would likely join. (All that is required is the placement of a placard and brochures in the waiting area.)

Because current informed consent practices often don't include explanations of how little is understood about the long-term health consequences of particular ART drugs or procedures, many women are not making truly *informed* choices. They don't know, for example, that one drug commonly used to suppress ovarian function—leuprolide acetate (Lupron™)—has never been approved by the FDA for this purpose.

Cracked Open candidly reveals the raw and debilitating physical, emotional, and spiritual challenges created by deeply personal and life-altering ART procedures. It will help generate a much-needed public discourse that could also become the clarion call for regulation of a field of medicine that has thus far unsuccessfully regulated itself.

Michele Goodwin,
Everett Fraser Professor of Law
University of Minnesota Law School
Editor of *Baby Markets: Money and the New Politics of Creating Families*
Author of *Policing the Womb*
Minneapolis

Judy Norsigian
Executive Director
Our Bodies Ourselves
Cambridge

ONE EGG, PLEASE, AND MAKE IT EASY

I am an official member of the *Late Boomer Generation*. We grew up after the Pill and the Baby Boomers, in the socially transformative 1970s and '80s, watching with wide eyes while millions of American women—some with children and some not—infiltrated formerly closed-to-females professions like medicine, law, and politics. This exodus from the kitchen into the boardroom created a thrilling, radical shift in home and office politics, in the economy, and in relations between the sexes.

"Shoot for the stars," some of the more thoughtful women advised us, "but don't forget about the kids."

We are the generation that also came of age at a time of burgeoning reproductive technologies. We grew up with dazzling front-page stories heralding the marvels of test-tube babies, frozen sperm, and egg donors; stories that helped paint the illusion that we could forget about our biological clocks and have a happy family life *after*—not necessarily before or during—the workplace promotions.

Each week newsstands brimmed with stories about older celebrities becoming mothers with the help of miraculous fertility treatments. A few years ago, photographer Annie Leibovitz *birthed* her first child at the age of *fifty-two*, while actress Geena Davis delivered at forty-eight and supermodel Christy Brinkley at forty-four. More recently we read about singers Mariah Carey and Celine Dion delivering twins at forty-one and forty-two, and actresses Courtney Cox and Marcia Cross became mothers at forty-three and forty-five, respectively. From where we stood, science and technology was the New God, giving women once considered over the hill a chance to start a family in middle age. Whether we knew it or not, we comforted ourselves in a security blanket of medical and media reassurances that age and motherhood no longer mattered.

❖

On my wedding day, a friend of the family asked if I was going to have children. I told her I didn't know.

"You're so young. You have plenty of time," she responded. "My sister-in-law never wanted children and she had two in a row in her early forties. You'll do just fine."

I was thirty-five at the time, but I wasn't worried about conceiving. I was more concerned about my ability to raise an emotionally balanced and healthy child who felt loved and respected. My soul had barely survived the second half of my own childhood and the idea of creating a family, now that I was finally happy in a relationship, seemed counterintuitive to me. I had true faith in my husband's parenting abilities, but when it came to me I still had serious doubts. I always needed to know there was a way out of whatever situation I was getting myself into, and I learned at an early age that children and exit strategies don't mix. Once a baby is delivered into your arms, you are its sun and its moon, its wheat fields and rivers. Without you, it will die. I looked upon this as an enormous responsibility and to some degree a great burden. Parenting was simply too overwhelming for me to consider—until the day I turned forty and realized that I would never be the Mother from Hell I imagined myself to be.

That morning, I *solemnly* swore that my number-one life priority would be making a baby. This courageous decision marked one of the first times in my conscious adult life that I intentionally placed all my eggs, so to speak, in one basket. That October morning, I looked in the mirror at the faint crows' feet visible around the outer corners of my eyes and gave myself a stern talking to. "It's time," I told myself. "No more flip-flopping on the baby issue. It's now or never. Understand?"

I meekly shook my head yes. I may have run away from motherhood before, but I was ready for it now. So five years after I had first uttered the words "I do," I said it again. I put my fears and arguments on hold, threw my birth control pills out the window, and tried to make a baby the "old-fashioned way." After six months and no pregnancy, my nurse practitioner suggested that my husband, Michael, and I begin using an ovulation kit. "It will tell you when you are ready to ovulate," she said, patting me reassuringly on the arm. "You can also rely on your vaginal discharge. When it becomes very viscous, like egg whites, you'll know you're ovulating or near ovulation."

Like so many other well-meaning people in my life, she was confident I would become pregnant. "My youngest child was born when I was forty-three," she said, beaming me a big smile. "You just never know."

Her faith in me meant a lot, and I began to latch onto the idea that I had invincible eggs and Michael had invincible sperm. I was optimistically convinced that together we could certainly make at least one baby. We hopped along the Baby Trail equipped with our little ovulation kit, going through the motions of intercourse as directed on the back of the box we purchased at CVS. On a certain day of the month, I would pee on the stick provided and when we saw the appropriate set of colored lines come into focus like an old Polaroid photo, we would stop what we were doing and make love. Fourteen days later, I would pee on a home pregnancy stick and wait for the right constellation of colors to appear, which they never did. Each month we waited with great anticipation that we might be pregnant, and each month we weren't.

One day well into the Baby-Making Process, I collapsed on the floor during a yoga class. Intense pain flooded my lower right side, and I became dizzy and nearly fainted. I managed to drive myself to the hospital emergency room where I received the first of many ultrasounds and vaginal probes. Tests revealed a cyst on my right ovary that doctors believed was endometrial. Bad news for two reasons: one, endometriosis was known to inhibit pregnancy, and, two, it was likely to become inflamed and irritated again during my monthly cycles unless I had surgery to remove it. While I was contemplating what we should do, pain once again dropped me to my knees. Eight weeks later, for the first but not the last time in my life, I was sedated while my gynecologist removed visible signs of the growth from my womb.

All in all, we had lost about six precious months of baby-making time, putting me at close to 41 years old. If I had been deaf to the ticking of my biological clock before, it was now so loud it kept me awake at night with worry. Though we were both wary of the medical establishment, everyone we spoke to told us that if we really wanted to have children it probably was time to weigh in with a S.W.A.T. team of fertility experts who might help us to conceive.

We chose a prominent clinic in the Boston area that, according to its website, was highly regarded in the industry for being one of the founders of IVF—in-vitro fertilization—otherwise known as the test-tube method of making babies.

Twenty years earlier, as a young newspaper reporter at the peak of my fertility, I had written an article about the first test-tube baby born in Massachusetts. The mother lived in my hometown, and I snuck into her hospital room claiming to be a family member. As I snapped a photo of the young woman tenderly holding her newborn, it was clear that she didn't care that her daughter had been born as a result of a then extremely controversial technology. She just seemed happy to be holding her tiny, healthy baby girl.

The article read, in part:

The Beverly Times, Tuesday July 25, 1984

KATIE'S A HIT IN TV DEBUT
By Miriam Zoll, *Times* Staff, Boston

Dressed in a pink polka-dot dress from Bloomingdale's, tiny Katie Louise Harwood, Massachusetts' first "test-tube baby," made her television debut along with her elated parents, Cathy and Doug Harwood, at Beth Israel Hospital.

Katie's two grandmothers and an aunt, who were visiting the Harwoods after the news conference, said they thought in vitro fertilization was a "fine" method used by couples unable to conceive naturally.

"It was nerve-racking because there were problems and you didn't know if she would be able to carry the whole term," said one of the grandmothers. "I don't consider my first granddaughter a 'test-tube baby.' It's a funny word, because it isn't in a test tube. It's a normal birth with different means of getting pregnant."

Two years ago the baby's mother, 26-year-old Cathy Harwood, had surgery to remove her right ovary and fallopian tube, and last February the doctors removed the other tube. "Right off we knew we'd have trouble," Doug Harwood said, sitting on his wife's bed. "We didn't have a choice—it was either this or adoption. We were down to the last option and we wanted children very badly."

The world's *first* test-tube baby had been born in Britain in 1978. By 2012, approximately 1.5 million assisted reproductive technology (ART) cycles were being performed annually worldwide, with an estimated 350,000 live births and 1,150,000 failed cycles (76.7 percent). In the United States, the *Fertility Clinic Success Rate and Certification Act of 1992* requires the Centers for Disease Control (CDC) to publish self-reported ART pregnancy "success rates" from the more than 440 fertility clinics throughout the country. With no standardized reporting mechanism, the rates are based on cycles that require manipulation of egg and sperm outside of a woman's body. They do not take into account success or failure rates of intrauterine insemination (IUI), hormone treatments alone, or donor cycles that abort. The CDC website states that a comparison of clinic success rates may not be "meaningful," because patient medical characteristics and treatment approaches vary from clinic to clinic.

"Success rates can be reported in a variety of ways, and the statistical aspects of these rates can be difficult to interpret," says the CDC.

"As a result, presenting information about ART success rates is a complex task…. Clinics do not report to CDC the number of women treated at each facility. Because clinics report information only on outcomes for each cycle started, it is not possible to compute the success rates on a 'per woman' basis, or the number of cycles that an average woman may undergo before achieving success."

Keeping this caveat in mind, by 2009, the latest year for which *full* data was available at the time of this publication, the CDC reported that 146,244 ART cycles were performed in the United States, and of those that used fresh non-donor eggs or embryos, approximately 63 percent failed. The overall number of live-birth deliveries for all ART cycles was 45,870 (32.4 percent), with a total failure rate of 100,374 cycles (67.7 percent). Overseas, the European Society for Human Reproduction and Embryology claims that 537,287 cycles were reported from thirty-three European countries including the U.K., the most active countries being France: 74,767; Germany: 68,041; Spain: 54,266; the U.K.: 54,314; and Italy: 52,032. Data from Japan show that in 2007 the total number of infants born as a result of ART was reported to be 19,595, close to 2 percent of all births.

◆

On the morning of our first appointment, Michael and I were nervous and excited. The clinic literature cited studies claiming, "Well over two-thirds of all couples seeking treatment for fertility-related problems become parents." It didn't occur to us then to ask if this statistic meant that two-thirds of parents birthed their own babies or a donor egg baby, or if they became parents through adoption or surrogacy. We were as green as could be about what to expect and what to ask, and we were eager to hear how the doctors thought they might help us.

We were also surprised at the number of young couples we saw in the waiting room. All along, we had thought older couples were the largest ART consumers. We quickly learned there was a growing trend of infertility plaguing younger couples that some studies linked to increased stress for women and exposure to environmental toxins, particularly plastics. A 2007 *State of Fertility* report issued by IntegraMed America Inc.—the nation's largest chain of clinics—indicated that the percentage of female college graduates between the ages of twenty-two and twenty-nine seeking ART grew by 23 percent from 1995 to 2002. It is not clear how many of these women are egg donors. Some research has shown that, for women under thirty, the chance of conceiving naturally in any given cycle is about 20 percent. Using ART, women under the age of thirty-five purportedly have more than a 30 percent chance of becoming pregnant, *which should never be confused with or compared to delivering a healthy newborn.* CDC 2009 data show that women younger than thirty-five are in fact the largest and most successful ART consumers (38.9 percent) in the U.S.

Across the globe today, an estimated 9 percent of women aged twenty to forty-four experience infertility lasting more than twelve months, and most who seek out ART are between the ages of thirty and thirty-nine. In most age groups in America, according to the CDC, percentages of ART cycles that resulted in live births were lower for women who had previously undergone an unsuccessful cycle. Data provided by the clinic we chose indicated that the "male factor" accounted for 35 to 40 percent of all infertility cases, compared to 20 to 25 percent from "unexplained factors," 15 percent from "tubal conditions," 10 to 15 percent from "ovulation disorders," 10 percent from conditions related to age, 10 percent from endometriosis, and 5 percent from uterine and cervical conditions.

That first day, we met with two health care professionals, one who examined my female interior and another who walked us through the ins and outs of the medical aspects of fertility treatments. A marble egg sat on a little pedestal on both staff members' desks, and at one point during our meetings they each held it between their thumb and index fingers. In the spirit of Vanna White, the former *Wheel of Fortune* hostess, they smiled and said, verbatim: *"Like we say here at the clinic, it only takes one good egg to make a baby."* It was obviously the clinic's mission statement. I immediately thought that, if all we had to do was find one good egg, we were certainly the right candidates for the job. How hard could that be, really? We had the best of modern science and medicine at our fingertips. I was in great mental and physical health. I exercised and practiced yoga regularly. I ate well. What more could a doctor ask from a patient? Little did I know that the process of finding one good egg would be a bit like panning for gold in a mine that had already been stripped of much of its bullion.

◆

A few weeks later, we met with a veteran physician I like to refer to as the Silver Fox. He greeted us with a warm handshake and a smile, and gave us time to look at his marble egg and photos of ferocious sperm fertilizing healthy eggs. Once he read through our medical records, he sighed very dramatically, clasped his hands together on top of his desk, and looked me straight in the eye.

"The first thing I want to say is that you're old."

I winced as his words cut through me like a razor-sharp sword, and then within a split second I found myself in a serious state of denial, fighting back the urge to tell him that he was the one with the white hair, not me. He was the old geezer in the room, not me. No sir, not me. All my life I had to convince people that I wasn't as young as I appeared. I knew I was teetering on the brink of officially entering middle age, but I didn't think I was there—yet. Sure, I noticed the sagging little pockets of skin forming beneath my chin and the heavy lines etching into my brow. I even acknowledged that the flab of my triceps had taken on new dimensions and that I might one day take flight. I knew all of these things already. I didn't need him telling me I was getting older.

"Women your age have a harder time conceiving, especially if they have endometriosis," he continued. "You should have come to see me when you were thirty."

Why thirty? My friend Sarah became pregnant the first time she tried at the age of forty, and Tracy got pregnant the first time she tried at forty, and then again at forty-three. Susan and Stephanie, my colleagues at the United Nations where I was working, both delivered without IVF at forty-two and forty-three. I was a little shocked by the doctor's recommendation, but I quickly learned that, after witnessing the failure of the technology time and time again, a growing number of fertility specialists around the world were now advising women to have their children in their *twenties.*

A few years ago, Susan Bewley, a respected British obstetrician, and her colleagues published an article in the *British Medical Journal* counseling women who wanted to have children to stop "defying nature" and do it before they entered their third decade. "If you want a family—and most people want a couple of children—and you are going to complete your childbearing by thirty-five and leave time for recovery in between, you would be wise to start before thirty," wrote Bewley, who specializes in high-risk pregnancies at Guy's and St Thomas Hospital in London. "Surveys of older mothers show that half say they delayed because they had not met a suitable partner. Maybe instead of waiting for Mr. Right they ought to wait for Mr. Good-Enough, if they want children."

As you can imagine, her comments caused quite a commotion, particularly among women who did have children after the age of thirty-five. Bewley was forced to publicly apologize on the website Mother35plus.com after she compared Britain's soaring teen pregnancy rate—the highest in Europe—to the "*epidemic* of middle-age pregnancies" that was also straining the national health care budget.

"The last thing I want to do is insult anyone," she wrote. "However, my colleagues and I have been concerned about the increasing distress and complications we are seeing [in older women]. There is a rising amount of infertility, miscarriage and complications of pregnancy as the average age of childbearing goes up."

Of course she and the Silver Fox were right. Older women do experience more complications, but did they really think that women just beginning to establish themselves professionally were in any kind of position to disengage from the workplace and the security of their paychecks? On top of that, did they really expect a whole generation of women to coparent with someone they didn't really love and risk the financial and emotional challenges that single mothers the world over endure?

When I was thirty, my writing and public policy career was just beginning to fall into place, and I *never* thought about my fertility. I was too busy working with a remarkable team of women producing the Ms. Foundation for Women's original "Take Our Daughters to Work Day." I was young, I wanted to travel, and I wanted to have *fun*. I wanted a life of action and corner offices. New York City was my ticket to living a life completely different from the one I had come from; from the one my mother had lived. Instead of looking for someone to marry and have kids with—something, by the way, that the majority of my women friends never thought about either—I set off on the path of proving myself in Manhattan. Like millions of other young American women just starting their careers, paying off student loans, and developing their confidence, I did everything I could to avoid motherhood. I used birth control like a woman possessed, squeezing half a tube of spermicide into my 1950s'-style diaphragm each time I used it. For the first time in my life, rather than just listening with envy to everyone else's exciting adventures, I finally had enough confidence and skills to travel and work overseas. And at thirty, I wasn't involved with someone I loved, let alone someone I *trusted* enough to have children with. There was no way I would ever settle for Mr. Good-Enough.

PUSH-ME, PULL-ME-LOVE

Mr. Right is my husband Michael and the story of how we came to be husband and wife is complicated. Our love is deep and our souls are bound, but our relationship over the last quarter-century has not been easy, which is one of the main reasons why we didn't have children when we were thirty, as Dr. Bewley and the Silver Fox advised.

We were acquaintances at university where I worked as an editor for the college newspaper. He rode his motorcycle about town, looking like Michelangelo's statue of David come to life. The first time I met Michael, I saw a vulnerable man-child who appeared to be perpetually windswept: some article of clothing always askew, a shoelace inevitably untied or a shirt untucked, and always a look of mischief and the joy of being alive.

I had moved to Boston after graduation and was compensating for my very meager income freelancing for the *Boston Globe* and the *Boston Herald* by cleaning houses. One day as I stepped off the curb at a busy intersection, Michael literally whizzed past me on his bicycle, missing me by about six inches. "Hey, watch it!" I yelled in a pissed-off voice, not knowing who it was. He turned around, saw me, and rode his bike right up to where I was standing. "Hey, Miriam. It's me, Michael," he said, with a big smile that could melt glaciers.

"Michael?" I said shyly, cursing my luck that one of the handsomest guys I had known at college was now standing in front of me while I was dressed like a bag lady. We chatted for a long time on a park bench about his recent travels to China and India and made a date for the next day. On Plum Island, we walked for miles along the beach and through the wildlife sanctuaries. We had been body surfing for only a few minutes before I realized that a wave had dislodged my bathing suit top and exposed one of my breasts. I was mortified at my discovery and looked to see if he had noticed. He had.

"It's been that way for ten minutes," Michael said with a big smile as he caught another wave. "It's okay."

Within an hour, we were out of the water and frolicking in the dunes.

"We're trespassing on the piping plover's nesting ground," I told him.

"No worries. We'll be careful not to squish them."

Our ocean date marked the initiation of an on-again, off-again courtship that lasted three passionate, tumultuous years. I was 24 years old and most of the time, for reasons you'll read about later, I felt panicked and afraid. In the darkness of the night while I slept in Michael's arms, I often felt compelled to leave his bed, upset at one thing or another that he had or hadn't done. Regularly at midnight, I would pronounce that the relationship was over and walk home alone in the rain or snow, pushing away the warm glow of his hands and his kisses. The love and attention he showered on me, at that time in my life, felt like the most threatening force on the planet. But like clockwork, the next morning I would show up on his doorstep with coffee and croissants, ready to begin our relationship anew. It would upset Michael when I'd leave his apartment so distraught. He didn't necessarily understand my need to run away, though he was *always, always* happy to see me when I returned. But this kind of push-me, pull-me love eventually ended our relationship and helped motivate me to begin therapy. Difficulties from childhood were now spilling over into my love life. I needed to make sense of it all. Eventually Michael and I parted ways, and I moved to New York City.

❖

I moved to Manhattan without a job. I was twenty-seven, around the age the Silver Fox and Dr. Bewley said I should have started focusing on my fertility and my desire to have children. Instead of entertaining thoughts of procreation, though, I was excited about the prospect of being swallowed up or mercilessly spared by the grinding wheels of capitalism and competition. I spent two weeks flipping through the Yellow Pages and calling newspapers, advertising companies, and public relations firms to see if they needed a writer. Much to my surprise, most of the people I spoke to were eager to meet with me.

An editor at the New York *Daily News* flipped quickly through my *Boston Globe* news clips and said she'd hire me for ten dollars a story.

"Ten dollars a story? How am I supposed to pay the rent?

"That's your problem, not mine," she said slamming my portfolio closed with a loud thud. "You either want the job or you don't."

I eventually found employment teaching creative writing in the New York City public schools. With no real training, I bravely rode the subway to schools in the Bronx where the classrooms were packed with forty-five or fifty students. I felt like a child myself, and my teaching stint lasted only a year. A perpetual survivalist, I discovered that I could earn fifty dollars an hour as a temporary secretary through Kelly Girl secretarial services. Relying on my extremely speedy eleventh-grade typing skills, I temped for some of the city's largest Park Avenue banks and law firms. With little time and effort I'd finish typing a full day's worth of client material in the morning hours and still have time left over to write plays and articles for myself in the afternoon. Over time I grew quite adept at switching back and forth between the client's data and my own writing. One morning I typed an important letter for an attorney while also perfecting a poem I had been crafting for my boyfriend.

"Are you done with that letter yet?" the lawyer asked me as he impatiently paced between his office and my desk.

"Oh, it's almost done," I told him cheerfully as I added the following new line to my masterpiece: *And you were like Beethoven playing classical notes on my pubic bone.* Right at that awful moment, he stepped directly behind my chair and started reading over my shoulder. Much to my embarrassment, he read the *entire* thing, then tapped me on the shoulder and said, "That's a great poem, kid, but I need my letter—now!"

"Yes, sir," I said, my face redder than beet soup.

At the time, I lived in an apartment across the street from the Williamsburg Bridge in Brooklyn. Though today that neighborhood is a trendy artists' community, back then it possessed a dirty, seedy quality that was oddly balanced by the surreal presence of a large Hasidic Jewish population known for dressing in black clothes and wearing felt hats. Back then, the intersection of the bridge and the East River was a place where prostitutes turned their tricks, and I was often approached and harassed on my walks home from the subway.

"I'm not a hooker, you schmuck," I'd yell, giving the finger to the men in company cars and vans searching for blow jobs.

At night the bridge glowed with shimmering white lights that reminded me of fireflies, and one evening I awoke to the sound of a woman singing. I crept to my bedroom window and saw the dim out-line of a petite young woman with dark hair who had nestled into one of the recesses of the granite bridge footings. Strung out on drugs or drunk, she kept losing her balance and almost tumbled several times onto the sidewalk. She wore white mid-calf boots with tassels like the ones high-school baton twirlers wear in Texas town parades. I spied on her for close to two hours before a car drove up and she somehow managed to drag herself to the passenger door and climb in. As the car sped away, I looked up at the night sky wondering how it was that fate had landed me in this warm apartment on a cold winter night while she had ended up out there. Life was a crap shoot, I decided, recalling the phrase, "There but for the grace of God go I." I thought of that phrase often as I walked through the streets of New York, and later, when I worked for the United Nations, roaming through cities in Africa where old women with leprosy and blind eyes begged for money.

❖

Several years had passed when I learned through the grapevine that Michael had moved to Manhattan to manage his uncle's just-opened Angelika Film Center. I was living with my photographer boyfriend in his loft in SoHo, and as far as I was concerned Michael wasn't allowed to set foot in *my* neighborhood. The Angelika—named after Michael's German aunt—was the hottest new movie theater in New York City, serving paninis and cappuccinos instead of popcorn and Coke. Convenient as it would have been for me to see films there, I avoided it for almost a year. I told myself I didn't care if Michael was nearby or not. I had moved on with my life. Some days on my way to work I would see him on a ladder changing the names of the movie titles on the marquee. I would always watch him from a distance but never spoke to him. As far as I was concerned, he was part of a past I had no desire to resurrect. Until one day when I was squeezing a grapefruit in the produce section of Dean & DeLuca, that museum of food for the rich and famous who live below 14th Street. With a Ruby Red in both hands, I heard a laugh so distinct it I knew it could only belong to one person.

"Oh no—Michael's here," I whispered to myself as I ducked below the fruit bin. I scanned the pastry and pasta counters, and then I saw him in line at the cash register with his sister. I reacted to the sight of him the way an ornithologist would study a rare bird, with excitement and intrigue. After that one-sided sighting, however, I was ruined. I became obsessed with running into him on the street. If I saw a man with dark curly hair walking along Broadway, I would pick up my pace to see if it was Michael. At the subway I sometimes wrestled my way through a five o'clock crowd so I could sit next to a Greek or Italian man who resembled him. Despite my militant denial that I didn't care,

I was obviously still intrigued. Finally, a friend convinced me to go with her to see a film at the Angelika by the remarkable Japanese director, Akira Kurosawa. Michael was working in the ticket booth.

"Why, Miriam! Hello," he said, using the same mixture of surprise and calculation that Cary Grant used with Katherine Hepburn in *Philadelphia Story*.

"Hi," I said tentatively. "I heard you were managing the theater now. How is everything?"

"Fine. Everything is just great," he said, looking me right in the eye while handing someone a ticket. "Why don't you find me after the show and I'll buy you a coffee, on the house."

"Presumptuous of him," I thought to myself during the film. "I haven't seen him in two years, or is it three, and he thinks I'll just cozy up to him over a cup of coffee. We'll see about that." I was so busy debating whether I should actually join him afterwards that I barely saw the beautiful images on the screen. Of course, when the film ended, I hurried upstairs and found him at the concession stand.

"Miriam," he said suavely. "How nice. Come, let's have coffee." Like a sultan ordering a platter of dates, he signaled one of the workers behind the counter to whip up two cappuccinos. We caught up on small talk and then I left, convinced that I would never see him again.

A few months later, I broke up with my boyfriend and moved into my own one-bedroom apartment on the corner of Ninth Avenue and 23rd Street. Conveniently, Michael had also ended his relationship with his girlfriend, so we were both ready for a reunion. Whatever bad blood had tainted our previous incarnation as a couple was not evident now, and we began spending a lot of time together. We cruised the city streets, gorged on caffe latte, and made love in the afternoons. His plan after one year at the Angelika was to move back to Boston to open a café. I would have preferred to stay in New York, but I loved Michael and knew we would have a good life wherever we decided to live. I was just happy as all hell to be reunited with him again.

When he finally did move back to Boston, I flew up only a couple of times before a mysterious woman from the former Yugoslavia whose name I am not allowed to mention arrived on the scene. *She* was from the same hometown as Michael's friend David S., whom he had met during his travels in Israel a few years earlier. The story I'd been told was that, in an attempt to be declared mentally unfit for military service, David spoke in tongues and bit off a chicken's head in front of a Yugoslavian commanding officer. In response, the military police beat him senseless and broke both of his arms and legs.

At some point in their friendship, David sent a photograph of Michael to *her,* and she supposedly fell in love with him based on the picture. For years, she used to send him postcards from exotic locations in Africa, Asia, and Latin America, where she worked for an Italian count as a hostess on safaris. She was also an accomplished equestrian and a first-class markswoman. Michael was apparently smitten by her James Bond-style resume and sultry European accent, because on one of my weekend visits to Boston he told me that she had visited him.

"She is Croatian," he told me as news clips of the Bosnian war flashed across his television screen. "Her home in Zagreb has been bombed. She's in the States temporarily on refugee status, but if she doesn't find a place to live, they will deport her. How do you feel about her staying with me for a while?"

A long time ago Michael had spent one night with this woman, who believed they were destined to be lovers for life. I was devastated that he was now asking me what I thought about her plan to move in with him.

"So, you want me to give you permission to let her live with you?"

"Well, what do you think?"

What I really wanted to say was that he was a jerk for even asking me. How could he possibly be raising this question after I had opened my heart to him a second time?

What I ended up saying was, "I can't tell you how to lead your life. It's your decision."

Needless to say, his question and my answer put a stop to our long-distance relationship. Back in New York I tried to figure out what had happened. As far as I was concerned, when you are in love with someone you don't ask a new lover to move in with you. What was he thinking? But as the months passed it became clear to me that I truly loved Michael and wanted to be with him. So on Christmas Eve I called to tell him that I thought it was ridiculous that we weren't together. When his answering machine picked up, it was *her* voice that I heard. I hung up, and a crushing sensation of loneliness and loss exploded through my whole body like a gasoline fire.

I had lost the love of my life, someone I thought had been my soul mate. How could I have been so mistaken about him and my own feelings? Six weeks after that fateful phone call, I telephoned Michael at his newly opened café. Luckily a woman with an American accent answered and asked me to hold. A few minutes later he came on the line.

"Hello?"

"Michael, it's Miriam."

"Oh. I'm really busy now. It's not a good time to talk."

"Yes it is. You're going to listen to me because after this conversation I am never, ever going to speak to you again."

"Okay," he said hesitatingly. "Go ahead."

"That woman you are now living with needs a green card to stay in America and she's using you to get one. You're going to end up marrying her, but you shouldn't, because you have no idea what love really is. You should never have children because people like you are the kind that mess their kids up."

In response to my advice he told me he loved her. "She is the woman of my dreams."

"I hate your guts and I'm never going to speak to you again," I told him as I slammed the phone down. I was shaking from head to toe. With tears streaming down my face, I stacked kindling and logs inside my beautiful brick fireplace and lit a match. Then I took out all of my photo albums and searched their pages for images of Michael and me. I burned each photo, one at a time, while chanting some kind of good-bye epitaph to him in between sobs. I extinguished every photograph except for the one of us sitting on top of a mountain with the sun shining down on the crowns of our heads.

❖

That July, Dudley Do-Right married his damsel in distress in a very elaborate wedding ceremony at a stone castle overlooking the Atlantic Ocean. While they exchanged vows, I became reckless. I started smoking more cannabis and drinking Cabernet Sauvignon every night. I dated men I did not like just to prove that love was stupid. I took personal risks I never should have taken, playing on the razor's edge and not even noticing if blood was trickling down my leg.

On my birthday a bouquet of yellow roses arrived on my doorstep. There was no card. When I called the florist to ask who had sent them, she told me the person had requested anonymity.

"If you don't tell me who sent these beautiful flowers, I am going to have to come down to your store and stage a sit-in."

"I can't tell you. It's confidential."

"Well, how about if I name some people who might have sent them. If I say the person's name, will you confirm if it was them or not?"

"Yes, I can do that," she said happily and we spent half an hour on the phone as I listed every person in my Rolodex. Michael's name was the last one I mentioned.

"It's not Michael Shashoua, is it?" I asked.

"Yes," she said with bubbling enthusiasm. "Yes, it is. Is that a good thing?"

"No," I said. "No, that is not a good thing."

I put the roses in a vase on my desk and stared at them. Though he had probably sent this gift as a peace offering, I interpreted his actions as a slap in the face. How typical of him to profess his interest in me *after* he had married someone else and to do it anonymously so he would not have to take credit for his actions.

"Fuck you," I said to the flowers as I packed them up in the box they came in and placed them at my neighbor's door, leaving her to ponder who had sent them.

❖

It was about a year after Michael's wedding that Sharon Gannon of the Jivamukti Yoga Center in the East Village initiated me into the world of yoga and I began a devotional practice that is still central to my life today. Often she invited us to dedicate our practice to someone we loved and, much to my chagrin, Michael's image frequently nudged everyone else out of the way.

"How could you, Miriam?" I'd berate myself. "He's married to someone else. He doesn't love you. He doesn't exist in your life anymore. Forget about him."

Regardless of the intellectual rationalizations, I couldn't let go of him. My subconscious wouldn't let me, and since yoga is about telling the truth, I decided to stop denying his spirit the space it still occupied in my heart. I devoted my practice to him time and time again while I dated other men.

Over the course of three years, I formed relationships with two retired NFL players (a linebacker and a quarterback who at thirty-three and thirty were almost crippled), a man who looked like Frieda Kahlo, a guitar-playing cowboy, and a French HIV/AIDS researcher who told me he didn't need to wear a condom because only drug addicts got AIDS. I also briefly dated a longhaired drummer who worked the nightshift at a bakery uptown making biscotti from midnight until six a.m.; when he became depressed he went for days without bathing. My therapist was astounded at how well versed I was at choosing unsuitable and unavailable men. Deep down I knew I was shielding myself from men who had the real potential to displace Michael's still dominant presence in my heart. I still compared every man I met to him.

One day my friend Melissa called and told me that Michael's marriage was on the rocks. "He's left Boston," she said in her Mata Hari informant whisper. "He bought a beat-up hotel and restaurant on the beach at Cape Cod. He's in pretty bad shape."

I was upset at this news. Despite everything that had transpired, I wanted Michael to be happy. He deserved to be sitting at a sunny breakfast table with daffodils and a plate of honey-butter and toast spread out before him. Instead, he and this woman from the land of vampires were fighting and screaming at each other night and day.

"They are miserable," Melissa continued. "He had to bolt his bedroom door to keep her out. It's a bad scene."

"And why are you telling *me* this?" I asked her.

"Because he still loves you, Miriam," she blurted out and then apologized for mentioning it.

"What do you mean?"

"He asked me not to say anything, but he knows he made a terrible mistake. He talks about *you* all the time."

A little smile of glory flashed across my lips. I was the forgotten prizefighter who had won the title after all. Except that I had no intention of ever going back to someone who had abandoned and mistreated me as deftly as he had.

"If he loves me so much why did he marry her?" I asked.

"I don't know, I don't know," Melissa kept saying.

And there it was. Michael's love had made its way back to me, but it was an unreliable love.

❖

Ironically, the third reunion between Michael and me again took place on the front steps of the Angelika Film Center. Just as I was arriving to watch a new Chinese film called "Raise the Red Lantern," he and his college roommate, Rick, were exiting the theater. When I saw him a circle of neon orange danger flags immediately sprung up around me but something told me to stand my ground. Since I had vowed that I would never *ever* utter Michael's name again, I called out to Rick instead.

The poor fellow turned around, tapped Michael on the shoulder, pointed at me, and then bolted away like a rabbit.

"Hello," Michael said, his hands in his pockets and his head slightly bowed.

"Hello," I replied, hovering above him on the top step like a fierce female warrior.

"I've been hoping I'd have a chance to speak with you, Miriam," he said in a very soft voice.

"Oh, really? Do you want to talk about how you fucked up my ideas about love or how you fucked up my life?"

"Oh, I think I would just like to talk," he said, realizing then and there that he would have to eat crow if he ever wanted to spend time with me again. "Can I take you to lunch?"

We went to Arturo's on Houston Street and talked for two hours over wine and pizza, and then we walked through SoHo on our way to a movie. In the elevator, Michael stared at me for what seemed like a very long time. That was when I realized that he really did love me and that his marriage had been a huge and terrible mistake. Even more illuminating was the fact that, after spending six hours with him, I didn't want to say goodbye. He was so familiar. After everything that happened, I felt like a chump but I also recognized and *honored* the deep feeling of relief I felt at being near him again. If there was one thing I had learned through the powerful combination of therapy and yoga, it was that pride and ego were disposable; the human heart was not. Love was only static if you boxed yourself in, and my yoga practice had taught me that walls could always be torn down. For me, seeing Michael again was like coming home, though I didn't let him know that for another few months. Technically, he was still married and I didn't want to get involved until he was divorced. When he left messages for me, I didn't return his calls.

❖

With fate and timing on my side, I began working part-time in Boston for Northeastern University's Center for the Study of Sport in Society. My friend Jackson Katz, now a leading international violence prevention educator, had just partnered with the Center, and they needed help launching his Mentors in Violence Prevention (MVP) program. The highlight of my time at Northeastern included meeting Mohammad Ali the night he was inducted into the Center's Hall of Fame. As the media coordinator of the event, I managed logistics for dozens of journalists and photographers who had come to see their legendary hero in person. That night the former heavyweight king and antiwar activist performed some magic tricks, played the piano, and later mustered up enough energy to walk up on stage to accept his award.

Michael called a couple of days later, and this time I answered the phone. "In case you're interested, I am now legally separated," he told me. "And I read about you being Mohammad Ali's spokesman in the *Boston Globe.*"

Spokesman? The media never gets anything right, but what a great mistake, really, to be connected to Mohammed Ali eternally in ink. I was proud of the misprint.

"How would you like to drive with me to Cape Cod to see the restaurant and hotel?" he asked. I hesitated, enjoying the thickness of my silence. A part of me still wanted Michael to suffer as payback for how I had suffered.

Then I said, "I'd love to."

That day I was introduced to more than the Oceanview Motel and Capers Restaurant, for that was also the day I met Luke. Michael had picked me up at the dingy apartment I was renting in Cambridge, and when we walked out to the street I asked him which car was his. He pointed to a blue Chevy Blazer.

"But there's a dog in the front seat."

"Yes," he replied nonchalantly. "That's Luke."

"*You* have a dog?" I asked incredulously. During all the years I had known Michael, he had never mentioned that he even liked dogs.

He opened the door and commanded Luke to get in the back seat but the dog just sat there looking at me and then at Michael and then at me again. He was mulling the situation over in his canine brain and wasn't quite sure what to do. If he could speak, I'm sure he would have said: "This is my seat. I always sit next to Michael in the front. *You* can sit in the back." It took a bit of prying and, when the seat was finally empty, I was accosted by millions of dog hairs that were stuck to the upholstery, the ceiling, and the steering wheel. In addition to the stray hairs, a horrific odor pervaded the vehicle.

"I'm not sitting there," I told Michael, who, like Sir Walter Raleigh, took off his jacket and spread it out on the seat to protect me from the canine debris. With snowflakes falling on the windshield, I breathed through my mouth the whole ride to the Cape.

Michael's seaside hotel faced the beautiful island of Martha's Vineyard. During the first couple of years, he managed to open in time for the tourists, but he could barely pay his monthly mortgage. The hotel was a cash cow, but since year one the restaurant and bar had been a black hole draining away all his profits. Initially planning to open an Italian seafood restaurant, he quickly learned that he had inherited a former rough-and-tumble biker bar. People still associated it with fistfights and police sirens on Saturday nights. In order to stay solvent, he soon replaced the Chianti and shrimp scampi with beer and fried clams. The day I arrived at this still broken-down ocean resort, he was preparing for his fourth season. Little did I know that I would spend five summers there.

◆

We were married at an inn on Martha's Vineyard. When the invitations were mailed out, friends in New York called to inquire if I was pregnant. They couldn't imagine that I would willingly enter into marriage unless I was knocked up, and they had reason to believe this. In my decades-long efforts to defend against my own fears of intimacy, they had listened to me pontificate about the historical roots of the institution of marriage dating back thousands of years to protect men's paternity and property rights, including ownership of women and children.

The reason I did marry Michael was because one day he gave me an ultimatum. He told me straight out that he wasn't prepared to stay in a relationship with me unless we were husband and wife.

"You're kidding—right?" I asked, thinking that he was damn lucky I was with him this very second considering the fact that he had gone off and married some war refugee five years earlier instead of me.

"No," he said, dead serious. "I'm not kidding. I love you. I want you to be my wife."

"I don't see why we have to involve the state and all our relatives in our love life," I grumbled. "Let's just live together until we grow old and die."

He shook his head. "It's not political, Miriam. I want you to be my *wife*."

I felt a flutter of fear and a rising sense of dread. I realized later that these emotions certainly had something to do with my trepidation about becoming someone's "wife"; I was deathly afraid that if I said yes I would seal my fate and enter into what I imagined would be a life of domestic drudgery, like the one I had watched my mother live. But I was also afraid of losing Michael again. Had we come this far in our reunion only to separate again because I didn't want to sign a piece of paper?

I was silent for a moment, and then I looked him in the eye and said: "All right. Let's get married."

◆

Shortly after our wedding, I developed an odd habit of suspending my work and social plans in order that I might excel at being a WIFE. My mother had taught me that being a good spouse meant having dinner on the table every evening at six so your grumpy husband and ill-mannered children could inhale their food with their grubby hands and never once thank you for the soufflé that didn't sag or the house that sparkled. From my reference point, the very definition of the word "wife" meant bondage; it meant never leaving the house, giving up your career, and never traveling abroad again.

After a week of witnessing me in my new role as a Stepford Wife, Michael inquired as to why I was so keen on cooking dinner every night, followed by an hour or so of housecleaning. "What are you doing?" he asked me.

"What do you mean *what am I doing?*" I replied. "I'm clearing the table."

"No, I mean what are you *doing?* You don't like cooking every night. You have other things to do. What's with the little apron and the Martha Stewart meals?"

I looked at him then, dazed and a little unsure about what I had assumed my new wifely duties were supposed to entail. "Isn't this what you do once you get married?" I asked with complete sincerity. "Don't you give up everything you've ever been or done and just stay cooped up in the house and cook and clean?"

"You do whatever the hell you want to do," he said. "You go to New York. You go to D.C. You work. You travel. You practice yoga. You write books. You don't just cook for your husband."

"You mean you don't expect that?" I asked incredulously.

"Of course not," he said with love in his eyes.

Though intellectually I knew that being a modern wife in the United States did not mean I had to be an indentured servant, on an emotional level I still didn't quite understand that an alternative existed. So many women in my mother's generation had sacrificed and silenced themselves in order to stay married to their Mr. Good-Enoughs. That night as the asparagus lay steaming in the pot, it suddenly dawned on me that Michael and I could have a liberating and expansive marriage; it didn't have to be stifling. I didn't have to be a martyr.

WELCOME TO CASINO FERTILE

Michael had known I was ambivalent about having children, but a few months before our wedding I brought the subject up again. With tears in my eyes, I told him that, if having a family was so very important to him, then perhaps we should rethink our relationship. I wanted him to know that I could not guarantee him parenthood. He professed his love for me anyway but to-baby-or-not-to-baby became the source of many fights over the years. He was always half amazed at my fierce resistance to having children, and half filled with sorrow knowing that my own family experiences had so deterred me from the possible joys of hearth and home.

When I finally told him I was ready to try he was exuberant.

"I knew you would change your mind. I just knew it," he said, smiling and giving me a hug. "I'm so happy you're finally ready."

I was confident that, since my mother had birthed me later in life, I would have no trouble doing the same thing. During our first meeting with the Silver Fox, I proudly told him that my mother had been thirty-nine years old when I was born.

"Just because your mother did it doesn't mean you will too," he replied. "Do you think there's a gene for birthing in middle age that your mother passed onto you?"

In response to that question, I distinctly remember that I blinked three times. Um, yes, think me an idiot, but actually I did believe that since mom had done it I could do it. Why would I think otherwise? For decades, the Sunday *New York Times* and *People* magazine had reported that it was possible to birth a baby later in life, and American pop culture is loaded with messages telling women that they can become pregnant when they are older. In the movie *Parenthood*, Mary Steenburgen and Dianne Wiest *both* play the role of older women who have no trouble birthing babies, and in *Father of the Bride*, a middle-aged Diane Keaton delivers a baby on the same day her 21-year-old daughter does. And Barbara Kingsolver's novel *Prodigal Summer* introduced us to Deanna Wolfe, a wildlife biologist who mates with a younger man and miraculously births a baby with no problems at the age of 46. Year after year, the headlines and cultural messages screamed out: "Relax and sit back. You've got science on your side."

But now this doctor was telling me that I might *not* have science on my side, after all. He was telling me that I had *deluded* myself with misinformation and false hopes about my own biology—and, according to global research, I am not alone. Studies conducted among college students in Sweden (2005), Canada (2010), and Israel and the United States (2012) all point to a pervasive lack of knowledge about women's fertility and overestimations of the success rates of reproductive technologies.

Of the 400 women and men surveyed in Sweden, only a small minority knew that women's fertility declined after the age of thirty, or that it rapidly declined in their late thirties. A full one-third of the Swedish men thought a woman's fertility did not sharply decline until after the age of forty-five. The Canadian study of undergraduate women found that "they significantly overestimated the chance of pregnancy at all ages and were not conscious of the steep rate of decline for women in their thirties." In Israel, where 4 percent of all children are born as a result of ART compared to 1 percent in the United States, college-age participants were "overly optimistic about women's capacity to conceive, not only naturally, but also with the aid of IVF."

In the survey of undergraduates in the United States conducted in 2012, over half of men and nearly 40 percent of women said they wanted to have their last child between the ages of 35 and 44. However, two-thirds of these women and 81 percent of men believed that female fertility did not markedly decline until after the age of 40. One-third of women and nearly half of men believed this marked decline occurred after the age of 44—an age at which an IVF cycle is least effective. A full 64 percent of men and 53 percent of women surveyed overestimated the chances of couples conceiving a child following only one IVF treatment. The study concluded that "the discrepancy between participant's perceived knowledge and what is known regarding the science of reproduction is alarming and could lead to involuntary childlessness."[6]

In 2001, years before these studies were conducted, the American Society for Reproductive Medicine (ASRM) launched an infertility prevention campaign that met with fierce criticism on a number of fronts. The advertisements featured an image of a baby bottle in the shape of an hourglass with text explaining how factors such as age, smoking, weight, and sexually transmitted infection can hamper future fertility.

The International Council on Infertility Information Dissemination said the ASRM's efforts focused too much on preventable infertility rather than on more serious conditions like endometriosis, polycystic ovarian syndrome, poor egg quality, inherited disease, and bad sperm motility. The campaign, they said, blamed the victim rather than the disease.[7] Kim Gandy, then president of the National Organization for Women (NOW), was quoted as saying: "Certainly women are well aware of the so-called biological clock. And I don't think that we need any more pressure to have kids." In an op-ed piece, NOW commended the ASRM for attempting to educate women about their health, but said their approach blamed individual women and their behavior for a more complex medical condition. "The ASRM gets free publicity," NOW said, "and women are, once again, made to feel anxious about their bodies and guilty about their choices."[8]

Still, I berated myself for being one of the those women who believed that technology had finally eclipsed Mother Nature and that my biological clock, in fact, didn't matter as much as it used to. A steady column of fear and sadness rose inside of me like a tidal wave about to hit.

"In a situation like yours," our doctor said, "where your hormones are not stimulating the kind of egg production needed for pregnancy, we like to recommend that couples think about egg donation or adoption."

"But we're not interested in those options, at least not now," Michael said calmly. "We know we are older than many couples trying to conceive but it seems as if a lot of them do succeed. Statistically speaking, what do you think our chances are of getting pregnant?"

"It's really random," the Silver Fox replied, this time looking right at Michael and holding his palms open in front of him like two empty bowls. "A successful pregnancy requires one good egg. We just don't know."

Making no promises, the Silver Fox invited us to roll the dice with him and we accepted his challenge. *You never know unless you try.* Instead of playing blackjack at Casino Royale we were now standing inside the gold-plated halls of Casino Fertile, a dazzling palace full of hope where we could gamble thousands of dollars as often as we chose for the *possibility* of scavenging for one good egg. At Casino Fertile the men in suits were doctors, the stakes were human life, and the perils were far greater than the guarantees.

❖

Each time we arrived for an appointment, the doctors and nurses made note of my age. This constant reminder of the passage of time accelerated my natural aging process more than any other event in my life. To feel vibrant, healthy, and sexy after forty is a good thing. I was still in my prime, according to me. But for those who probe the deep interior of the female body, I was well over the hill and categorized as premenopausal. When friends came for dinner and asked how I was, I told them I was doing okay considering the fact that I was an Old Hag. The depression had already set in. I aged considerably in mind and body that year. All my former life successes scattered in the wind and dissolved into nothingness, the way the Wicked Witch of the West melted into a puddle of green ooze. I was just a sack of wrinkled skin and brittle bones. Nothing mattered anymore. My eggs were old.

❖

My parents dispensed medicines to us kids and took us to the doctor when absolutely necessary, but more often they espoused a holistic approach to treating illness. If we had a cold, we stayed in bed and drank lots of fluids. If we had a sore throat, we gargled with salt water and sucked on a Sucret. Michael and I adhered to a similar approach to healthcare, choosing old-fashioned remedies over pharmaceuticals on most occasions. But when it came time for us to decide whether we would venture into the world of test-tube babies and high-tech drugs— or risk not having a child at all—we went against our instincts and chose the drugs and procedures.

Each time we began what is referred to in the fertility industry as a *cycle*, I received a prescription for birth control pills. Though it makes no sense to the layman, ingesting the Pill enabled the White Coats to monitor and control my endocrine and reproductive system to such a degree that they could calculate pretty close to the exact moment—or so they claimed, and I believed them—when I might ovulate. Clinic nurses taught us how to inject very expensive hormones—often $5,000 for one round—like Follistim, Ganirelix, and Luveris into my abdomen. Early on, we decided it would be best if Michael administered the drugs so that he could play some kind of role in this bizarre conception process.

"I hate this," he'd say, pinching my stomach flesh between his fingers and swabbing it with alcohol. "I hate to think of what these drugs might do to you ten years from now."

"Don't think about it," I reassured him, "I'll be okay." But I worried about it too. Very few medical studies had tracked the relationship between potent fertility drugs and the health of women undergoing treatments, including egg donors and surrogates. Several studies I had read talked about increased risks of breast cancer and ovarian tumors, and some made links to cancer and developmental delays arising in children born from some technologies. But for every study that claimed a connection, there was another one that said there was nothing to worry about. There was no conclusive evidence.

"I need to position the needle just right so that it goes in straight and not at an angle. If it's angled, it will bruise you."

"And hurt."

"It will be okay," he'd say cheerfully. "We're going to make a baby this way. Maybe two." Then I'd nod my head, take a deep breath and close my eyes as he plunged the syringe into my belly.

On the fifteenth day of our first cycle, I went to the clinic for an ultrasound to determine if the drugs had stimulated any follicle growth. Using a vaginal probe that resembled a fat, white plastic penis, the technician scanned first one and then the other ovary searching for ripe eggs. The most precious follicles measured somewhere between eight and twelve centimeters. Like a good laying hen, I generated five eggs on my first cycle, and this pleased the doctors. If the eggs thrived they would then be *harvested* from my ovaries and fertilized with Michael's sperm. If the embryos sustained healthy cell division of seven cells or more, the clinic staff would then *transfer* them into my womb. Even though I knew some ARTs evolved from veterinary medicine and the desire to breed better thoroughbreds and other livestock, I must confess that when I first heard this fertility lingo, I was a little taken aback. I was a woman, after all, not a chicken. People who ran fisheries and poultry farms harvested eggs. I was in love with my husband and for the first time in my life maternal instincts were keeping me awake at night. Was the clinic staff really going to harvest my eggs? In my mind's eye, the doctors and nurses lined up in a single row like the Rockettes at Radio City, nodded their heads simultaneously, and sang out: "Yes, that is exactly what we're going to do."

On Harvest Day, the nurse escorted me into the operating room and laid me out on the gurney while the anesthesiologist filled the veins of my left arm with sleeping potion. I actually enjoyed the sensation of slipping away and waking up an hour later with no recollection of time passing. Poking a long needle through the walls of my vagina, the medical team extracted the five good eggs from my ovaries. Meanwhile, upstairs, Michael was in the sparsely decorated Ejaculation Room where all the men who already feel useless in this process go to spill their seed. Michael has confessed many times that one of the most difficult things he has ever done is jerk off into that tiny cup knowing that two floors below I was lying unconscious on the table, my pelvis hoisted to the ceiling, like a cow at a slaughter house.

After they fertilized the eggs, the embryologist carefully watched for cell division. Two days later, all but one embryo had ceased to exist, but the remaining one divided into seven cells—a decent number. It might just be our *"one good egg."* We promised each other that if a baby resulted from this hocus-pocus we would name it *Siete,* the Spanish word for the number seven.

The day of the transfer we were very upbeat, smiling at each other and stealing kisses. The attending nurse looked at us and asked if it was our first time.

"Yes," we both responded enthusiastically, our white smiles dazzling in the sun.

"Oh" was all she mustered in reply before she slumped away.

We donned our very unfashionable but sterile hospital garb and padded into the operating room. This time no anesthesia was necessary. The cherished embryo was placed inside a catheter that was then inserted into my uterus. Using ultrasound to scan the interior of my womb, the attending physician nudged the tube ever so gently, depositing the embryo to flourish or to die.

❖

We spent the next two weeks monitoring my breasts and abdomen for detectable traces of tenderness and swelling. The clinic finally called to tell us the pregnancy test had come back negative. We were shocked. We had been absolutely convinced it was going to work.

Until this point we had both assumed that *other* people had trouble getting pregnant, but us—well, we were something special. We were supposed to get pregnant on the first ART and then send the doctors on their way. But as dazed and disappointed as we were by the failure of the technology and my biology, we headed right back to the clinic for another round of talks, medications, and ultrasounds.

This time the Silver Fox prescribed an alternative cluster of drugs and suggested we actively work to reduce our stress load.

"Try some yoga and meditation," he advised.

"I'm a yoga teacher," I told him. "We both practice yoga."

"Good," he said. "The less stress in your lives, the better your chances."

Unfortunately, he didn't warn us that this new hormone cocktail's side effects had the potential to transform me into a menacing amalgamation of Attila the Hun and Kathy Bates's character in Stephen King's thriller *Misery*. After several weeks of this emotionally turbulent drug regimen, the results of the ultrasound indicated that it was time once again to harvest my eggs. I donned the ugly hospital gown and shower cap for the second time and walked stoically into the operating room. As the cold liquid of the anesthesia flooded through me, I vaguely remember hearing music that one of the staff had kindly piped into the room with his new iPod. The attending physician was dressed in black that day, like Johnny Cash, and I drifted off mumbling the words to "Folsom Prison."

When I woke an hour later, a young doctor was kneeling by my bedside. He took my hand in his and said, "I'm sorry. We only found one good egg this time. I'll pray for you." I was still foggy from the sedation, and he faded from view like a FedEx messenger leaving me with an empty box of hope. In the mist of half-consciousness, I began to panic. My ovaries weren't responding to the drugs. The insurance company was paying for only some of these procedures, and our out-of-pocket expenses were mounting. Maybe we should enter one of those bizarre IVF raffles that clinics had started offering in states like Texas and New York. Devastated contestants plumb out of cash enter the contest by submitting emotionally charged stories about their uphill battles to conceive. The "winner" receives a free cycle, and the clinic receives a public relations boon that supposedly boosts business. The real question for us was: How many procedures would it take until we got pregnant? How many could we afford? Would any of them actually succeed? I suddenly realized that those middle-aged celebrities on the cover of *People* and *Us* may have actually endured multiple cycles and spent hundreds of thousands of dollars before they posed for the camera with their little bundles of joy in their arms.

Despite my fears, *Uno*, as we called this lone embryo from our second cycle, sprouted mightily under the nourishment and encouragement of Michael's sperm. Needless to say, we were elated when they transferred it into me on a Thursday. Sadly, Uno did not cling to my womb either.

❖

With our emotional denial growing stronger every day, we rebounded through the second failed cycle and assumed that our chances of finding that one good egg would be even better on the *next* round of potent drugs. We had no reason to believe this. At a follow-up meeting with the Silver Fox, he suggested once again that my age was a huge disadvantage. Statistically speaking, he said we had a 2 percent chance of conceiving with my eggs, and there was no guarantee that such eggs would produce a healthy child. At this stage in the game, we needed to worry about Down Syndrome and other genetic disorders. Once again, he suggested we consider a donor egg.

"What exactly does that entail?" Michael asked.

"We retrieve healthy eggs from a donor between the ages of eighteen and thirty-two, fertilize them with your sperm, and transfer them into Miriam's womb," he explained matter-of-factly. "Miriam's uterus nourishes the embryo, her amino acids help build its life structure. The baby would have her blood. Miriam would be the birth mother."

With telepathic exactitude, Michael and I looked at each other and silently mouthed the words, "I don't think so."

❖

Entering into the world of assisted reproductive technologies is a bit like traveling to another planet. The process challenges you to reassess everything you thought you knew about yourself and the world. All the loose ends that took you decades to tie into a nice, neat package called your life are suddenly untied again. Long-held beliefs about right and wrong begin to flake off your psyche like old paint on a windblown house. Moral dilemmas about eugenics and cloning become common themes in your midnight dreams. You find yourself actually considering what it might be like to create new life, not just in a Petri dish but also in a Petri dish with *someone else's eggs*.

A year ago the idea of using a stranger's egg to make our baby had been unfathomable. But now? Now we were seriously starting to at least investigate it as an option. I had thought we were two very down-to-earth people who admired the mystery and power of nature, which we considered divine. If that was true, then what were we doing talking about creating a baby with Michael's sperm and someone else's egg? I was revolted by our desperation.

"It's just an egg," Michael said nonchalantly one night.

"Then why don't you just put an ostrich egg inside of me?" I retorted.

"It's just one cell."

"It's someone else's cell. It's someone else's life history and someone else's ancestors. It's not me."

"But we might not be able to make a baby with your eggs."

"Maybe not, but I'm not putting someone else inside my womb. Why don't you just mate with the donor instead and take the baby once it's born? Then I don't have to go through a pregnancy knowing that I'm carrying someone else's child inside of me."

"It would be *our* baby," he said softly. "Half me, one quarter her, one quarter you—and you would be its mother, not her."

Whatever. I had issues with donor eggs.

There was the case in 2005 of the South Korean stem-cell researcher Hwang Woo-suk, who was deified by the international science community for being the first to extract stem cells from a cloned human embryo. He resigned from his post after admitting he had coerced and paid twenty of his junior female scientists $1,400 each for their eggs. His race for glory and, legitimately, for medical cures had interrupted his ethical censors. He fell from superstar status to leper in one day, and South Korea—and numerous other countries—has since categorized buying human eggs as an illegal act.

Despite my disparaging sentiments, the fact that I might have a better chance of bringing a pregnancy to term with donor eggs was nothing to balk at.

❖

"How many IVF cycles are we going to try?" Michael asked me one morning. "I mean, we could do this for years. I hate to say it but I think we are turning into fertility junkies. As long as we keep paying, the clinic will keep looking for our one good egg. We could do this dance forever."

Maybe he was right. My friend Mary and her husband endured *eighteen* fertility treatments in one form or another, starting when she was thirty-five and ending when she was forty. Their reproductive nightmare included multiple hormone treatments followed by three failed intrauterine treatments, otherwise known as IUI, whereby sperm is artificially inseminated directly into the woman's uterus at a very high speed. Though the success rates are lower in older women especially, many insurance companies still require that patients undergo this cheaper treatment before moving on to more expensive procedures. Mary then suffered through close to a *dozen* IVF cycles, three of which resulted in pregnancies that ended in miscarriage. By the time she walked away from the fertility boxing ring, she was more holograph than human; only the shell of who she once was remained to be seen. In the end, they adopted two baby girls from a prominent agency in Texas.

"Adoption is the only *guarantee* that you will end up with a baby in your arms," she told me after I confided in her that my first two cycles had failed.

"Have you tried donor eggs?" I asked. "I hear there's a good chance of conceiving that way."

"Oh yes, we tried donor eggs," she said with great wisdom in her voice. "That didn't work either. Adoption was the only guarantee for us."

Every time I'd bring up the subject of adoption, Michael would say that he had not yet given up on the possibility that we might conceive a biological child. As for me, I was quite certain that I didn't want to dedicate the next five or ten years of my life living a Fertility Fantasy. The invasiveness of the needles, the drugs, and the stirrups were a great strain, and the idea of being pregnant when I was older than forty-five was too strange to contemplate. The big question was: At what point do we accept nature's decision? At what point do we give thanks for all the abundance we have in other parts of our life and move on?

These were difficult questions to answer, and we kept finding ourselves in front of that wall that inevitably appeared and against which we inevitably beat our heads. We took turns asking ourselves if we had been so brainwashed by the West's exaltation of science and technology that we actually believed that these men—for most of our fertility doctors were men—could ignite life in me the way Michelangelo's painting, *The Spark of Life,* depicted God giving life to Adam. When push came to shove the answer was yes, we did believe that the doctors just might have that power. It was worth another try. We were so tangled in our web of desire and denial, so clinging to the notion of birthing a child, that we would gamble whatever emotional and financial capital we had and do whatever the doctors told us to do.

I took comfort in knowing that we were not alone in our frustration with our dedication to procreate. Watching the Nature Channel one night, I learned about the giant tortoises that spawned on the beaches of Costa Rica. Every year, they would have to contend with marauders and high tides as they laid thousands of eggs along the coastline. Only a small fraction of the tiny tortoises that hatched would make a beeline for the sea and thrive. It was that way for millions of mammals, birds, reptiles, fish, and insects struggling to conceive and safely birth their offspring. Human infants that withstand the miraculous journey of conception to birth often die too soon from hunger, drought, disease, or war. And some, like me, wonder how it is that we remain whole—in body, mind, and soul—when our family life has been less than idyllic.

JESUS CHRIST—OY VEY

Mary Baker Eddy, the founder of the Christian Science religion, believed that genuine healing was rooted in one's belief in God. In poor health and physical pain most of her life, she experimented with alternative therapeutic modalities and finally turned to the Bible in 1866 to explore the medical wisdom of the teachings of Jesus Christ. A decade later, the controversial Eddy published her seminal work, *Science and Healing with Key to the Scriptures*, which mapped out the main theological and curative systems that underpin the practice of Christian Science, also known as the Church of Christ. In 1881, she founded the Massachusetts Metaphysical College to pass her particular brand of healing on to others. Her disciples—Christian Science Practitioners—included doctors, lawyers, businessmen, homemakers, and my maternal grandfather, George Peck Bonney.

Born the son of a prominent Massachusetts physician, my grandfather ultimately surrendered any allegiance he may have had to his father's country doctoring and began instead to espouse the teachings of Christ. I have always wondered why the doctor's son became so adamantly set against medicine. Perhaps as a boy in the farm towns of western Massachusetts he had witnessed too many hacksaw amputations or wept at the sight of a child trampled to death by horses. Or perhaps it was due to his own and medicine's powerlessness to prevent the early death of his first wife, Elizabeth, who was miserably afflicted with muscular dystrophy.

The few photographs I have seen of him depict a tall, bald man with penetrating eyes who always wore a fedora and a jacket and tie. Relatives have told me that he was the kind of man who, even if his throat were parched, would offer his last sip of water to someone else dying of thirst. During the Great Depression it is rumored that one day he removed his shoes and socks and gave them to a homeless man wandering the streets of Boston. In exchange for his spiritual healing, he was often paid with a bag of potatoes, a basket of autumn apples, or a fresh-baked pie. Given this paltry income, his much younger second wife and former Sunday school student—my sassy grandmother, Marion—became the principal breadwinner in the family. At a time when most women did not venture outside the home, she and her sister worked for close to two decades as the proprietors of the Marigold Tea Room in Salem, Massachusetts, dishing up lamb dinners with mashed potatoes and fresh green beans for thirty-five cents a plate. In addition to earning an income when most women didn't, Marion was actively engaged in various clubs and guilds and was an accomplished poet, and, though she may never have called herself a feminist, I certainly would.

My mother, on the other hand, was a quiet and shy girl—a result, I think, of having been raised by an older preacher father who believed that children should be seen and not heard. She grew up in a quaint seaside cottage in a neighborhood known as the Willows, a place that exploded in the summertime with a rich, honky-tonk nightlife famous throughout New England. Back then, the well-greased train system of the Boston & Maine Railway delivered hordes of vacationers to the numerous hotels and restaurants that dotted the coastline. As the sun went down, the dance halls and saloons filled up with tourists eager to spend their money and laugh at the moon.

On the other side of town, my Orthodox Jewish father spent his childhood in skirmishes with the French Canadian Catholic kids whose families migrated to Salem to work in the mills. His Russian parents had arrived in America in foul-smelling passage ships at the dawn of the twentieth century, intent on building a new life free from the bloody religious persecution of the czar and his Cossacks. My grandmother, Lena, was a proud, illiterate woman who, according to my cousins, possessed a mean streak that often made their mothers cry. My Aunt Dottie once told me that Lena's tendency to hurt others stemmed in part from the fact that she never stopped loving the boy from her village who did not make the passage to Ellis Island as he had promised her he would. Though her heart longed for him she married and eventually grew to love my grandfather, Samuel, who pledged to love and protect her. He ran a successful haberdashery and kept the family well fed and clothed until the day his appendix burst and he nearly died from the infection. His recovery entailed sitting motionless in a chair for one full year staring with glazed and glassy eyes at the four walls of his bedroom. Though the toxins that flooded his body didn't kill him, my grandmother's rage at the loss of the family's economic security hung over him for the rest of his life. He later opened a cobbler shop where Yiddish-speaking Russian men used to congregate in the afternoons to gossip and drink whiskey.

Two years after he graduated from high school, my father enlisted in the Air Force, joining 16 million other military personnel who served their country during World War II. Black-and-white photographs from an old musty album show a handsome young man cavorting with street children in India and sitting under palm trees on the Pacific Island of Tinian. It was there that he once spied the Enola Gay, the B-29 that dropped the atom bomb known as "Little Boy," on the Japanese city of Hiroshima. Dad regrets never having had the chance to fight against the Nazis, but he did spend a considerable amount of time clashing with the ignorant southern rednecks in his platoon that called him names like "Kike" and "Jewboy." At a time when six million European Jews were being gassed to death, I'm sure it was painful for him to always be defending himself against attacks from his fellow Americans. By the end of the war, my gregarious and charming father had adopted a certain mistrust of the world. It seemed to me that he made up his mind that, since he was a Jew living in a dangerous world, life would always be hard and he would always have to watch his back.

Franklin Roosevelt's decision to sign into law the Servicemen's Readjustment Act—more fondly remembered as the G.I. Bill— enabled my father to earn a college degree at George Washington University after the war. It was during his pilgrimage home to Salem in 1950 that he discovered my beautiful mother sipping a Mai Tai in the Hawthorne Hotel Cocktail Lounge. In her stylish clothes and chic hairdo, she looked so much like the movie star Ingrid Bergman that people used to stop her in the street and ask for her autograph. They made a handsome couple driving through the WASP-y towns of Boston's North Shore in my mother's shiny Studebaker convertible. My parents picnicked and swam in the sea during the summer months and skied down New Hampshire ski slopes in the winter. But when they looked into each other's eyes they realized that despite their love the odds were against them: mixed-faith marriages were frowned upon in postwar America. To make matters more difficult, my father's family was still grieving over the atrocities of the Holocaust and could not find it within their hearts to condone their son's love for a minister's daughter.

In spite of the opposition on the home front, my parents continued an on-again/off-again relationship for eight years before they finally married. Their union was contingent upon my thirty-five-year-old mother agreeing to convert to Judaism and raise her children in the Jewish faith. A devoted lover, she studied the Torah and the Hebrew language and married my father in August 1958 at a synagogue in Boston. The day she said "I do," she left a trail of Christmas trees and Easter bunnies behind her and closed the door on her former life and self.

❖

Before she married my father, Mum had enjoyed two decades of social autonomy and economic independence working as a secretary in Boston. That life all but evaporated by the time she turned forty and spent her days juggling the chaos of caring for three children under the age of four. She devoted any additional free time to trying to transform herself from a Christian into a Good Orthodox Jewish Wife and Mother. Mum skillfully managed the logistics required for maintaining a kosher home, including keeping two sets of dishes and silverware— one for milk and one for meat—and even went so far as to learn how to make *challah* bread and to soak and salt beef. She stopped eating many of the delicacies she had grown up with, like scallops and shrimp, bacon and ham, or a dessert of ice cream or cheesecake after a nice steak dinner.

I remember that, when the pharmaceutical company my father worked for relocated him to Pennsylvania, my parents used to pine to be back in New England near family, friends, and the ocean. I sensed my mother's melancholy and loneliness, in particular. Dad went off to work every day and came home brimming with stories about coworkers and clients, but my mother stayed home alone trying to figure out which laundry detergent was best for removing grass stains. Though a job outside the home most likely would have boosted her spirits—and alleviated some of the ever-present financial strains my parents faced— they modeled rigidly-held traditional gender roles for their kids. In my family, the man was clearly the breadwinner, and the woman was expected to stay home, and that was just the way it was. As a result, over time my mother's former confident, income-generating self dissolved into that of a classically isolated housewife dependent on her husband for grocery money and a bridge to the outside world. Sensing all of this, I realized at an early age that a job with a decent income was everybody's ticket to freedom, but that for a female it was an indispensible lifeline.

All this old-fashioned behavior was pretty confusing to me. While my parents were busy recreating scenes from *Fiddler on the Roof*, my friend's mothers—and women across America—were taking to the streets demanding their right to control their reproduction and to access male domains like law and medical school and the U.S. Congress. I desperately tried to make correlations between the ladies talking about women's rights on television and the lady in the kitchen making dinner, but they didn't seem like the same kind of women and, in fact, they weren't.

My mother was born just three years after the Nineteenth Amendment granted women the right to vote. She was an entire generation older than these feisty Baby Boomers. Her family background and the era of the Great Depression in which she grew up had prepared her for a passive life of conformity, free of protest or overt rebellion. Despite the excitement of the revolutionary social and political changes occurring in the United States at that time, my parents' household continued to function within a framework of anachronistic gender norms and strict religious observances. The nuances and undercurrents of their marriage made it quite clear to me that I was living in a patriarchal—certainly not a matriarchal or egalitarian—family system.

❧

I have always believed that my father was wracked by enormous guilt for falling in love with a Gentile. Somewhere deep down in his subconscious he felt that his decision to marry my mother had made him a traitor to his faith and to his parents, who had endured such awful religious persecution in Lithuania and Latvia. He filled this gaping hole by inflicting Orthodox Jewish studies on his three children five times a week for more than a decade. Motivated by guilt and obligation, his fixation on molding his children into Good Jews eclipsed any prospect of actually sharing and exploring the spiritual beauty of an ancient faith with his offspring.

Many people muddle through and some even enjoy the monotony of their religious training. I found mine horrendously oppressive, claustrophobic, and hypocritical. While my friends spent their afternoons at swimming, dance, or horseback riding lessons, I was forced to sit in dingy classrooms that smelled of mothballs, listening to old immigrant men with hairy earlobes and bad breath talk about burning bushes and the persecution of the Jews. After being cooped up in public school for six hours all I wanted to do was ride my bike and feel the wind in my face. But when we kids voiced our frustrations over the rigors of

Religious Boot Camp, my parents made it clear that there was no room for negotiation or even discussion: Dad's guilt and Mum's need to conform meant that for years on end we had to suffer through Hebrew school three times a week *and* attend Friday evening and Saturday morning services. I was literally trapped in this nightmarish routine from the age of six until I was confirmed in the eyes of God at sixteen and officially released from bondage.

Though outsiders looking in may have thought they were witnessing benign discord between parents and children over religious studies, there was a much deeper subtext at play. My parents' decision to veil my mother's former life as a Christian meant that we kids were caught in a confusing net of hypocrisy; on some level we were pawns in an experiment to prove that *Mixed Bloodlines Could Produce Good Jews*. My parents may have tried to fool themselves into believing that a few blessings from a rabbi could erase my mother's *goyish* roots and mannerisms but I knew better: Mum went through the motions of being Jewish but she was always a Gentile to me. From my vantage point, it seemed that she had converted to Judaism in order to marry my father, and *not* necessarily because she was so drawn to the teachings of the Talmud and the heroics of Moses. As a kid, when I used to watch her pray in temple and light the Sabbath candles at home, I always thought she was pretending to be Jewish. There was a very theatrical and surreal quality to the religious charade that composed the central theme of life in my parents' home. There was a price to pay, too. I grew up thinking that my mother was an imposter and that my dad was trying to trick everyone into believing his family was something that it wasn't. As a half-breed, I never understood why we couldn't just be honest and tell the truth.

❖

As time and the challenges of parenting marched on, my father began to rule over his wife and children like a dictator with a devotion to his own desires. Though he has apologized many times since and carries deep regrets, on bad days his behavior illustrated an utter lack of understanding of the principles of democracy, equality, and respect for individual needs and differences. It is for this reason that I unfortunately associate a vast majority of my childhood with the era of communism in the former Soviet Union. Under the political and gender systems that he—and my mother—devised, the mundane dictates of my father's agenda took precedence over all others, and transposed the vibrant colors of liberty and the pursuit of happiness into the grayness of dull conformity and fear. My mother's inability to orchestrate a *coup d'état* of any magnitude offset the hopes we kids may have had for jumping ship and defecting. It was her inability to challenge my father and defend us from him that made me wary that, if I ever had kids, I would desert them the same way I felt she had deserted me. That was an unforgiveable offense and something to be avoided at all costs.

My dad employed a wide range of psychological tactics to keep his family in line, including guilt, humiliation, and manipulation. Sadly for my brother, Dad viewed his first-born son as an extension of himself and placed expectations on Danny that had nothing to do with who he really was as a person. Even as a small boy it seemed that on an almost daily basis my father berated Danny and his budding sense of self for one alleged offense or another. Dad exhibited an abnormal interest in Danny's masculinity and resorted to shaming him if he did not perform well in traditionally male domains, such as sports. At Pop Warner Football games he would harshly admonish him in public for dropping the football or would accuse him of hitting a baseball like a girl. Once when Danny and I were helping him build a storage cabinet, Dad became *furiously* frustrated with the way my brother was using the screwdriver.

"Don't turn the screw like a girl," he'd say as his face turned red and his voice rose. "Use the tool like this."

When I inquired if, because I was a girl, I'd never learn to do it right either, my father looked at me but never said a word.

His obsession for his son "to grow up to be real man" took a toll on Danny as early as elementary school, when he started wetting the bed. This is a common occurrence among children—particularly boys—and is often linked to an immature bladder system. Most children who suffer from this ailment cannot control it and are often terribly embarrassed and upset that they can't. In some cases—and I certainly believe this was true for Danny—the condition also develops in response to circumstances in the child's emotional life and home environment. Though mental health professionals advise against it, roughly one-third of parents—including mine—attempt behavior modification by punishing and shaming the child.

Unfortunately, rather than trying to alleviate Danny's own sense of humiliation, my parents choreographed a daily ritual that I believe devastated his dignity and only exacerbated and prolonged the problem. Most mornings for a period of six or seven years they crept into his room like two detectives investigating a crime scene. Looming like giants above him, they would wake him from slumber and draw the covers off his small body. If he had wet the bed—and he often had—my father unleashed a tirade of hurtful insults while my mother stood by his side mute as a statue. This still-painful episode in my life taught me that, contrary to what I had been reading in my fairytale books, not only stepmothers but actual fathers and mothers could inflict pain on children. It also made me realize that some mothers were just as powerless as six-year-olds who could not or would not protect their children.

The fact that my father was not always harsh with his children made his explosive outbursts that much more frightening. Many times he laughed and played with us for hours on end, and would let us jump off his shoulders at the lake or the pool. We'd scramble up the front of his body like spiders climbing a ladder and then count to three and dive or cannonball into the cool water. We had no idea why he changed so often from being a fun dad into a mean or irritable dad, but I always assumed it was due to financial worries and poorly managed stress.

I remember that in response to these unpredictable moods my sister, Rachel, and I used to close our eyes tightly at night in the bedroom that we shared and wish and wish with all our tiny might that Danny wouldn't wet the bed the next morning. We believed in magic, you see, and we thought that if we prayed hard enough our collective wish might somehow protect our brother. Most of the time it didn't.

Some mornings I would creep out of my room and peer through Danny's doorway only to see him lying helplessly in a pool of urine as my father's anger and insults pierced his tiny soul. With evident shame and humiliation in his voice, I would often hear Danny condemning himself for being a Bad Boy and promising that he would try harder next time. The ironic sick twist to this story was that no matter how hard Danny may have tried he really couldn't control his bedwetting: it was something he had to outgrow both physically and emotionally.

In adolescence Danny turned to drugs to alleviate his inner troubles, and later his addictions led to a three-year-long prison sentence for dealing cocaine to an undercover cop in the parking lot of an abandoned mall. Today he still feels daily the pangs of job discrimination and social stigma based on one poor decision he made when he was twenty-three years old.

❖

We moved back to the Massachusetts seacoast when I was in the sixth grade, into a dilapidated house with peeling turquoise paint, rotting porches, and an outdated interior. The best thing about it was its proximity to the beach: the ocean was only a three-minute walk away. I smelled salt air every morning when I woke up and every evening before I went to bed. From the moment we moved into that house, the beach became my new best friend and the refuge I sought when I needed to escape the chronic fighting and tensions at home.

By junior high school Rachel had begun holing up in her bedroom where, she recently told me, she was incredibly depressed. Like Danny, she was also heavily entrenched in warfare with my father. Ever the addict for conflict and control, Dad had literally forbidden her to date the Catholic boy who lived down the street.

"You married a non-Jew," she'd scream at him. "How can you tell me to break up with him because he is a Christian when you married a Christian? Your logic makes no sense. Just leave me alone!"

Of course my father didn't leave her alone. He responded to his elder daughter's request by stalking her. Like a crazed lone wolf, he would cruise the streets of our town banging on Rachel's friends' doors to inquire if they had seen her. Then he'd drive to the beach or a nearby park and shine a flashlight beneath bushes where he thought she and her Gentile boyfriend might be frolicking. Just as my parents' remedy for Danny's bedwetting only made matters worse, my father's constant bullying made Rachel dig her heels in even harder. Under more peaceful conditions, she likely would have quickly tired of this particular boy, but she grew closer to him instead. For four long years she fought with an admirable iron will like some great heroine in a Jane Austen novel. As the battles wore on, her personal power grew, and she learned how to stand up for herself in a way that I never did until I was much older. To some extent, the stress of her boldness and determination compromised her health and ignited a chronic case of colitis—and later two bouts of cancer, now in remission—that did not dissipate until she left home to go to college.

As the youngest child and a bystander, I was too immature to join forces with or rescue Danny and Rachel from their skirmishes with my father, and for that I will always feel a twinge of remorse. As I grew older, I tried to defend them verbally, acting as their defense attorney time and time again in a family courtroom that usually ignored any relevant evidence I may have presented. When the bullets began to fly I learned to move out of the line of fire, but I still absorbed the impact of the dysfunction the way a second-hand smoker inhales other people's toxic cigarette smoke. Like my mother, I cultivated my own quiet way of coping. I did not turn to drugs like Danny or openly rebel like Rachel. I became bulimic, committing acts of violence against myself in the camouflage of night.

Controlling what I put into my body and what I expelled seemed to be the only way I could register any sense of jurisdiction over my own life. In therapy years later, I came to realize that, for me, vomiting had little to do with body image and much more to do with expressing silent, frustrated screams of anger. That was partly why coproducing the original Ms. Foundation for Women's "Take Our Daughters to Work Day" had been such an important project for me; the campaign's original theme was "to make girls visible, valued, and heard." When I finally told my parents years later that I had been bulimic, they were speechless. They were either in shock, thought I was crazy for doing such a thing, or felt enormous guilt about it. We haven't talked about it since.

LIFE AND DEATH

When Michael and I recovered the hope we had lost after the second IVF cycle failed, we bravely advanced to our third. Despite all the medical evidence stacked against us, we were trying to maintain an upbeat and optimistic attitude.

"What do they know?" Michael would say, trying to boost our spirits and keep us from drowning in our diagnosis of infertility. "They can't guarantee the outcome in either direction, so why not try?" And he'd rally me, coaching me that if any couple could pull this off we could. It was a mind game that just might work.

Knowing how stressful the treatments were for couples, the clinic offered a whole counseling component to complement their medical services. In the late spring, I called to sign us up for a ten-week couples support group that cost several hundred dollars. Organizers claimed that half the participants ended up conceiving, while also learning to enhance communication skills and reduce stress. It sounded good to us. Much to our amazement, an apologetic receptionist called back a few days later to tell us that, since there weren't enough people signed up, they were not going to convene the group.

"But the social worker and the doctors have been recommending this to us," I explained. "They think it might help us conceive."

"I'm sorry," she said.

"What this is really about," Michael said to me angrily when I told him what had happened, "is that there isn't enough revenue from just two couples, so to hell with us."

I had to agree with him. For months the clinic had been marketing the support group to us, and now here we were, struggling to keep our heads above water, and they were closing the door in our face. Once again we experienced the heartless side of the industry. But still we marched onward.

During our third cycle, we were introduced to Lupron, a drug that, depending on its dosage, can be used to either boost or repress estrogen production. Since I was *craving* personal space and freedom during this cycle, I was determined to learn how to plunge the needle into my own belly. Mastering the art of injecting a syringe full of hormones into your own body is not an easy thing to do. One friend of mine who traveled during a cycle spent two hours on the telephone with her husband while he tried in vain to coach her to self-inject. In the end, they had to abort the whole cycle, losing both precious time and money. Ultimately, Mission Stab Myself was successful, and Michael ushered me off to meetings in New York with an ice cooler packed with $5,000 worth of drugs, alcohol swabs, and needles.

I stayed with my friend Meryl, who was two months pregnant at the time. Like me, she had married a man who enjoys brief visits to Manhattan but has no desire to live there full time. Though she kept a small apartment in the city, her new home base was now Manchester, New Hampshire—a city that comes to life every four years for old-style presidential primaries and politicking. In the off years, the abandoned brick mills on the edge of the Merrimack River that once employed thousands of laborers now serve simply as monuments to an economic Golden Age long since gone. As anyone who has ever lived in New York and loved it can understand, it was hard for Meryl to adjust to life in the Granite State and to drive a car with a license plate that said "Live Free or Die." Once her beautiful son, Elias, was born, she jokingly referred to his nursery as "Cellblock E" located in her home in lovely downtown "Manchganistan."

One evening I was sitting at the kitchen table in Meryl's 13th Street apartment with my cache of vials and needles spread out before me. I was worried that someone looking in the window from across the street might think I was a heroin junkie.

"Can I watch?" she asked, obviously fascinated. This was the same woman who had photographed and later published a book about first-year medical students dissecting their very first cadavers.

"Sure," I said, glad for the company as I swabbed my belly with alcohol.

"How do you do it?"

"Well, first I fill the needle with Ganirelix. Then I push a tiny bit out so I don't kill myself with an air bubble. Then I hold a big roll of fat between my fingers, inhale, and stab on the exhale." Bam. The deed was done, and I had clearly earned her admiration. I like to think that, because I self-injected, I truly claimed the reproductive process for myself during that third cycle, surrendering any residual doubts I might have had about becoming a mother. I like to think that, because I self-injected, I became pregnant for the first time in my life at the age of forth-three.

I knew within a week of the transfer that we were pregnant because, like billions of women before me, I felt that my nipples were volcanoes burning hot with molten lava. The first night I noticed it, I woke Michael at two a.m.

"What is it?"

"It's my boobs," I said to him.

"What about your boobs?"

Surely he could see them glowing in the dark.

"My boobs are on fire. I think we're pregnant."

Having ridden the roller coaster of the first two cycles, Michael was more skeptical than I was.

"We should wait for the pregnancy test. It could just be hormones, you know."

"That's a fine thing to say to a woman whose boobs are burning up," I said under my breath, but he was already fast asleep.

I stayed up the rest of the night wondering if I would be this uncomfortable for the next nine months of my life. A week later, the clinic called and confirmed that we were indeed pregnant. We cried with relief and anticipation. Now what? Having lived a nomadic life, primarily in New York and Boston for close to a decade, we now started discussing how we really needed to decide which city to live in.

"You can't schlep a baby all over the place," I said. "A baby needs a stable home."

We talked about possible names and Michael said he liked the name Ramses, like the Pharaoh the actor Yul Brenner played in *The Ten Commandments*. If it was a girl, we liked the name Matilda. We discussed sleeping arrangements, schedules, day care, and nannies. We talked about how we would rig up a system for the baby on the boat so we could still go sailing in the summer. We made plans to expose the child to the world through trips to Italy and South America. We vowed that we would turn off the TV so the child could think for itself. We talked about all of this and more, and then floated into the ultrasound technician's office for our first post-conception examination.

Most of the ultrasound technicians I have met are not very talkative. They sit in a dark room all day long looking at a computer monitor as they meticulously track the microscopic movements of cell growth. Such work seems to require intense concentration, which leaves no room for small talk or even pleasant conversation. On this visit, I realized that these technicians are the first health care professionals to assess the health of an embryo and its heartbeat, the first to identify a cyst, or the first to measure a cancerous growth. Michael and I had been cooing like birds for a month, and now we were going to see our baby's heartbeat, the first photographs. We asked questions, of course, as we always did. What's this and what's that? That's your uterus. That's the zygote. That's the heartbeat. Right there, thumping on the screen we could see the heartbeat. Ping. Ping. Ping. We beamed at each other. Who knew we would actually make a baby?

A few minutes later, the Silver Fox met us in the hallway and invited us into a tiny office with no window.

"The heartbeat is weak," he told us once the door closed.

"What do you mean by weak?" Michael asked.

"It should be 160 per minute. It's only sixty. That's not a good sign."

Emotional denial seeped in under my skin.

"Who asked you?" I said silently to myself. "What do you know anyway? Ramses is a strong embryo. He'll get stronger. He just needs more time."

We found all kinds of excuses to keep the possibility of miscarriage away from our little bubble of a world. After all these years of trying naturally and then going through IVF, how could it possibly be that we were being told our embryo was in danger of never being born? We were crushed. Like tiny people thrown to the ground by giants we shattered into a million pieces. We had thought the hardest part would be *getting* pregnant, not *staying* pregnant.

"You'll miscarry within a week, most likely," he told us as he left the office.

Michael and I walked to the car in silence. At home, we immediately searched the web for information that might contradict the doctor's diagnosis. We did find a number of sites that said things like: "My baby's heartbeat was weak until the eighth week, then it increased to 100, then 120, then 140." Another site said, "Older women having children should disregard what the doctors say about heartbeat readings in the seventh week. My sister was forty-six when she had her first child and its heartbeat was eighty at the ultrasound reading. The next week it soared to 120. Her son is three today." The Internet is filled with websites and chat rooms geared toward older couples trying to conceive. Many of the sites provide heartfelt stories and testimonies of women overcoming the odds, and how they purposefully kept the medical establishment's dire predictions on the far back burner of their mind's-eye while they pushed forward with all sorts of alternative remedies.

One book that a friend gave me described a forty-three-year-old mother who was trying to conceive a second child. Two of the New York City IVF clinics she went to refused to even admit her as a patient because of her age. Finally one clinic did accept her, but they were pessimistic about what they might be able to do for her. In the end, she decided to forgo Western medicine and turned instead to acupuncture, nutrition, yoga, and other forms of exercise. The black ball landed randomly on her roulette number and she birthed a second child at the age of forty-four. But what works for one woman doesn't necessarily work for another. Fate, nature, and the chaotic theories of chance and randomness make more sense to me now. Getting pregnant is a crapshoot, and I was still losing all my chips.

❖

That evening I woke around three a.m. and went into the living room to cry. I cried and I cried and I cried. This new life we had worked so hard to conceive was shriveling inside me, its heartbeat fading with each passing hour. The convulsive sobs emanating from deep within my gut did not subside. I could not control them or conceal them from Michael, who wandered out of the bedroom and stood in the darkness with me.

"I don't have any comfort to offer," he said numbly. "I'm sorry you are hurting, but I have nothing in me to give right now. I am so sad."

So I spent the night emoting noisily on the couch while he burrowed deep inside himself, curling up like a caterpillar in our bed, insulating himself from the deep disappointment and sadness that gripped him.

❖

It is truly a fine art to learn how to focus on the potentially positive outcomes of a pregnancy rather than ruminate over the possibility of fetal death. Thinking optimistically when the odds were desperately stacked against us required that we simply put on blinders and charge forward in the most optimistic manner possible. Michael and I are extremely hopeful people to begin with and we never imagined that I wouldn't carry to term. I am sure that the couple at the clinic who kept us waiting for our doctor for over an hour never thought they would miscarry either. She was six months pregnant when she was forced to deliver her stillborn child through what must have been one of the world's saddest labors.

If a miscarriage has a sound, it is the deadening reverberation of a very heavy iron gate closing forever. On one side of the gate there is the life cycle, bright sunshine, flowing waterfalls, and the regeneration of plants, animals and humans. On the other side lie death and the universe and all of its black holes leading into the vast nothingness of billions of galaxies that exist beyond the tiny one that we occupy. Miscarriage reminds us that life is fragile and finite. It teaches us that presumptions of victory hold no weight in comparison to the powers of nature and fate.

Our miscarriage occurred at the same time both of our fathers were suffering from ill health. Their failing bodies made Michael and me much more aware of the proximity of death and of our own mortality. I spent many sleepless nights wondering whether, if we ever did become pregnant, either of our fathers would be alive to hold their new grandchild in their arms.

Fertility treatments taught me to see life as a board game. External rules were imposed. A certain amount of money was involved. I was told to advance. I was told to retreat. Sometimes it felt like I was winning. Most of the time it felt like I was losing. Without the proper mindset I might fall off the board game altogether, end up in the river without a paddle, even drown when no one was looking. It felt like a form of psychological torture. At night I would lie awake and replay the what-ifs and the should-haves of my life so far. I knew this game of replay was a sure sign that my youth was fading. I had never had regrets about my life until now.

Sleeping became difficult again, and the ticking of the clock roared in my ears like ocean waves at the height of a menacing hurricane. Images from my past flashed across my mind like a movie looping over and over, buzzing in my psyche like a plague of bees that refused to leave. I experienced a morass of emotions. There was rage accompanied by a deep, hollow hurt. I was angry that my body did not produce eggs. I was raging at a childhood long gone that still clawed at me and tried to drag me back in time. I was like a broken porcelain doll that had been glued back together, but the pieces did not line up in quite the same way. One eye was now lower than the other, one nostril higher, one leg longer. I was out of sync, out of sorts. I was Humpty Dumpty's buddy.

Michael and I often spoke about feeling broken. When his divorce finally came through, he had been so emotionally exhausted that he would limp rather than walk across the street. I told him that I hadn't felt this discombobulated since Danny went to prison and Rachel was diagnosed with cancer. I'd been piecing myself back together for twenty years and now it felt as if I was busted all over again. I was acutely aware of the fleeting flash of a lightning bolt, that one millisecond when the rain hits the pavement, the moment when a fetus' heart stops beating. Flatline. Flashes of time, the propulsion forward, and I couldn't stop the energetic momentum of life. I was in a surging ocean. I could only keep kicking with the movement of the water, with the current that almost drowned me.

❖

During the brief time I was pregnant, my father suffered a mild stroke. Having survived three cancers, he was now, at the age of eighty-three, lying in a hospital bed in large part because he had argued with his physician about taking high-blood-pressure medicine. She had told him he could either lose weight or take medication, and he did neither. He wasn't about to give up the crackers, pretzels, ice cream, and cake that he ate like there was no tomorrow. Over the years, I had tried multiple times to introduce him to diets that focused on volume control and carbohydrate reduction, but he only half listened as he chewed his second bagel and cream cheese of the morning.

"I like to eat," he'd tell me. "You can't teach an old dog new tricks. Leave me alone."

Standing beside his hospital bed with the fetus growing inside of me, I wondered if I should tell him that I was pregnant. What if he died tomorrow? He would never know that he would have been a grandfather for the second time in his life. If I did tell him, it might revive his spirits and give him something to look forward to. But, like millions of couples, we kept the news to ourselves, knowing we would announce when we were safely through the first trimester.

❖

Accepting death's nearness in your life is something that I think comes only with age. A typical thirty-year-old will usually not wake up at four a.m. because she's dreamed about burying a parent. It is when we grow a bit older that the idea of death settles into our psyche and seems to stay for good. It isn't as if you are fixated on it. It simply lingers there in the background, like a bodyguard sticking close to a rock star or a president.

Death became a permanent fixture in my psyche when Michael's Aunt Janet died of breast cancer. What had begun as a backache turned out to be breast cancer that then metastasized to her bones. For four long years, she courageously endured round after round of brutal and debilitating chemotherapy treatments. And then one day at Yale Hospital in New Haven she went away. Her soul lifted up and out, leaving the shell of her body on the bed. Just like that. Poof. Such an experience changes you forever. It is like you have seen into another dimension that you know exists but that you cannot define. The knowledge of death is like a fine fabric scarf that drapes ever so lightly on the skin of your face. You know it is there but you can't necessarily touch it or wipe it away.

◆

The path to parenthood through scientific means is littered with booby traps filled with snakes and burning oil. To keep from falling in, couples must be very dedicated to nurturing the love that bound them in the first place. If one member of the team stumbles and falls, as will inevitably happen, the other person must be there with an outstretched hand. I don't think many couples embarking on this path think about their chances of miscarrying. If they really studied the statistics and the medical journals, they would never set foot in an IVF clinic. But the fertility industry sells hope to couples distraught over their inability to produce offspring, and hope is a multi-billion-dollar business.

LIVING ON THE WILD SIDE

Michael and I have each exhibited nomadic tendencies since childhood, but it is also in our genes. He descends from a long line of Babylonian desert dwellers that wandered the dry lands of Persia for centuries via camel caravans. My ancestors were sea captains who skillfully sailed the vast oceans until the winds deposited them safely on the shores of Massachusetts, Hawaii, and Africa.

When we actively began trying to conceive a child, we decided that our wandering ways would no longer serve us once we became parents. Shortly after New Year's 2000, we decided to call a semi-truce to our never-ending battle about whether we'd settle in Boston or Manhattan. We were rabid loyalists to our respective cities: I felt that Boston was too stiff, and after three days in New York Michael couldn't handle the frenetic pace. During one of our many two-career/two-city geographic debates, he argued against Manhattan on account of the War of Independence.

"I will never live in New York City, or anywhere in the state of New York," he pronounced vehemently one day. "Do you know why?"

"Yes, you've told me a million times. Manhattan is crowded, it's expensive, there's no parking, and it smells."

"Not only that," he said with passion building in his voice. "New York sided with the British. They supported the Tories. The Tories! Boston was the antithesis of Tory."

"Give me a break. Are you really going to sit there and denounce the greatest city in the United States because they sided with the red-coats 200 years ago?"

"You bet I am. And don't forget that New York also had slaves. Boston was the bastion of abolition before it even became a movement."

"Boston had slaves, too. I can't believe you're stooping this low," I replied, exasperated.

It took a few months before we agreed to remedy the situation by purchasing a house in the rolling hills of western Massachusetts, roughly halfway between the two urban centers. Since we were both self-employed, the plan was that, as needed, we would travel to our preferred city a few days a month and the rest of the time we would nest and raise a family in the country.

We searched for a home in the foothills of the Green Mountains, roaming between Amherst and Northampton. This community is known for its beauty, its artistic cultural scene, and its educated five-college demographic. We finally hit upon an old, rundown farmhouse, complete with an outhouse, a chicken coop, two barns, and lots of land. Since Michael is a designer and builder, we knew that over time we could make it beautiful. That spring we made an offer on the house, and through a bizarre series of twists and turns we lost it. Miraculously, six months later it came back on the market and we closed the deal in less than two hours. We celebrated with a bottle of champagne at a friend's house, noting the uncanny parallels between finding, losing, and then securing that house and finding, losing, and finally reclaiming our love.

The morning of our home inspection was a lovely September day. The sun was shining on the fields and mountains across the street, and the sky was a perfect blue. The house, built in 1826, gave us more square footage of living space than anything we could ever afford in the city. As we were waiting for the home inspector and the septic engineers to arrive, our broker zoomed into the driveway with her car radio blasting. With a voice filled with panic, she informed us that a plane had just crashed into one of the towers of the World Trade Center. She and I manned the TV news coverage, providing tragic updates every fifteen minutes to Michael and the home inspector as they surveyed every inch of the old house. Within hours all of our lives, the face of our nation, and global geopolitical tensions had shifted. When we stepped across the threshold of our new house a few weeks later, it was a bittersweet moment. We knew we were also crossing into a new era of human history, which would be marked by more intense terrorism and hatred toward the United States. We interpreted our being safely together in the country on the morning of September 11, 2001, as a sign—an omen, really—that we made the right decision.

❖

It would be inaccurate to say that, after two decades of urban living, country life was a picnic. Like Captain Kirk and Spock in an old *Star Trek* episode, Michael and I beamed ourselves down into an environment unlike any we had ever experienced before. There was no high-speed Internet, no all-night bodegas, and no Chinese restaurants to deliver dumplings at two in the morning. There literally was nothing but mountains, grass, and stars. We thought there was no better place for us to try to get pregnant.

The first year that we lived in the house, neither Michael nor I ventured out to the driveway at night. There were no streetlights, and it was terrifyingly dark. When we opened the door, Luke barked at some invisible creature with fangs and claws that we couldn't see but that might actually exist. We lived in the region of the country that boasted the largest black bear population east of the Mississippi. Our neighbors had found moose tracks next to their car. Someone else thought they had spotted a bobcat, and, believe it or not, neighbors up the street— also transplants from the city—one day discovered a bear in their kitchen. Martha and her husband, Satch, had been watching television in their downstairs den when she heard a noise upstairs. Thinking it was just the cat knocking something over on the counter, she ignored it. But when the racket persisted she crept upstairs and saw a bear eating her freshly baked muffins out of the pan. It had swiped its way through the screen door with a heavy paw and apparently had no intention of leaving.

"I ran like hell to get Satch," she told us, "and we went out the side door to the car. We honked the horn and honked the horn and eventually the bear came out onto the back porch. But he took one look at us and went right back inside to continue with his feast." They spent ninety minutes in the car while the bear had his way with their house.

Our home, on the other hand, became a haven for small animals and insects. We had squirrels in the attic, snakes in the basement, and ladybugs so thick on the south-facing windows that you couldn't see sunlight streaming through them. When the squirrels invaded, Michael donned special anti-rodent battling gear—a hard hat, mask, safety glasses, and a thick shirt—to combat the 21 flying squirrels that squatted in the crawl space above our bedroom. Behaving as though they were on steroids and cocaine, these seemingly benign creatures thumped, crashed, and raced above our heads, making it impossible to sleep. The stench of their living quarters, coupled with a leaking slate roof, eventually filled the bedroom with such a noxious odor that we had to sleep downstairs for six months. In the end, poor Michael, a kind, nature-loving man, executed the squirrels, either by setting traps or smashing the not-quite-dead ones squarely on the head with a hammer. As horrible as the squirrel season was, the rats that came later will go down in history as one of those classic tales of country living.

They raided the house one month to the day after our beloved dog, Luke, died suddenly in the twilight of a hot July day. Being a city dog, Luke did not adjust well to the incessant sounds and scents of the various life forms that lived in and surrounded our house. Equipped with superb canine eardrums, he would wake us up with his baritone watchdog bark at all hours of the night, regardless of whether the wind blew or a raccoon passed by. Shortly after we moved in, I went to New York for a business trip and when I called home to check in I could barely hear Michael over the incessant noise of Luke's agitated barking.

"Is everything okay?" I practically screamed into the phone.

"Baby!" Michael said. "You won't believe what is happening here."

"What's going on?"

"The whole house is surrounded by a pack of howling coyotes. They want to get at Luke and he is pacing from room to room and barking. His hackles are up and his eyes are blazing. I've never seen him like this."

Our old farmhouse had been neglected for some time before we bought it. The grass around the house and in the fields across the street had grown to waist level, providing a perfect hiding area for coyotes, bears, skunks, raccoons, and porcupines. To alert the wildlife that there was a new alpha male in town, neighbors had recommended that Michael and our male visitors deposit their testosterone-infused urine around the perimeter of our property, and they happily obliged.

Luke spent much of his last year of life hunting small rodents and sleeping on the front porch. He was a good dog, a cross between two very seminal historical figures. In his great warrior dog moments, Luke was imbued with steadfast bravery like that displayed by Geronimo, the famous Native American freedom fighter. His more pampered Louis XIV side was most pronounced when he stepped into the shower with us demanding a bath and a blow-dry, or when he lay on his back, front paws lifted, waiting for us to rub his belly and scratch his ears. While he was with us in the country, Luke's very presence in the house did much to ward off the critters. I swear the night he died they all knew he had passed away.

Within days, our kitchen filled with rats. At first we weren't quite sure if the clues they were leaving behind belonged to large mice or some other kind of rodent. Like everyone's house on our road, ours was also infested with mice. When we discussed our mouse concerns with neighbors, they once again told us to get used to it.

"That's country living," they'd say, shrugging their shoulders and scratching their heads, as if to say, "What do you folks expect? You live in the country. There's always going to be mice in your house."

One day we came home and found scat on the kitchen counter and a bar of soap on the floor bearing teeth marks.

"I wonder what did this," Michael mused as he examined the vandalized bar of soap. The marks could have been made by any number of rodents that roamed our house, including mice, moles, or voles, those small blind creatures I often saw bumping into the baseboards as they made their way back down into the ancient fieldstone cellar. When we first moved in, I was awfully proud of that basement. It was a remnant of the true spirit of the New Englanders who had dug the pit and then carried the stones that formed the foundation of the house 160 years ago. I took pride in the fact that it was still intact, and I was fond of showing it off to visitors. But as the rodent and occasional snake and jumbo-sized salamander problem escalated, I began to resent the gaping holes that were obviously easy-access tunnels.

Though we retaliated against the half-eaten bar of soap by baiting more traps, we continued to hear noises in the walls while we ate our breakfast or tried to sleep. One week, we were both away and I returned home first. I had developed a habit of sneaking in the front door very quietly so I could listen for any mouse activity. On this particular afternoon, I heard a rustling in the kitchen so I tiptoed over to the doorway to listen. When I clapped my hands and stamped my feet, voilà! Up and out of the Cheerios box on top of the refrigerator popped a rat. It was a big rat with a big rat nose, the kind of rat I had just seen in Central Park in New York. The creature was very nimble as it scampered down the metal grill on the back of the fridge, descended into a hole in the floor and then escaped through the damned fieldstone sieve of a basement.

Of course I couldn't wait to tell Michael.

"You'll never guess," I said smugly when he answered his phone.

"What?"

"You will never guess what was in our kitchen. It was huge."

"Are you okay? Where are you?"

"I'm at the house."

"Is there a bear in the kitchen?" he asked, alarmed, thinking of Martha and Satch.

"No. It was not a bear. I kind of wish it had been a bear. It was a rat. A goddamn fucking rat."

"Are you sure it wasn't a mouse?"

"I'm sure it was a rat."

Silence. Then chuckling.

"I'm going back to New York," I told him. And I did. I walked out to the driveway, got in my car, and drove back to Manhattan.

❖

I had no stomach for exterminating rats. When push came to shove, I could set a trap but if it malfunctioned and the creature lay wounded I became so upset I had to leave the house. Sadly, the executioners' job fell to Michael who dutifully went to the local hardware store and bought the largest snap traps available. He baited them with peanut butter and placed them strategically in the basement, the kitchen, the garage, and the barn. He also bought rat poison and sent a communiqué to the entire neighborhood warning them to keep their dogs and cats away from our house.

"We-ah killing rats in these he-ah parts," he proclaimed like a true Yankee. At times like these, I often expected to see one of his front teeth falling out as he sucked away on a corncob pipe. My elegant, city-bred husband was turning country right before my very eyes and, though he was successful at trapping some of the rats, there always seemed to be more. We were up to a casualty count of six, I believe, the day I decided to roast butternut squash in the oven. I had turned the stove off an hour earlier to let the squash cool and had just taken a plate down from the cupboard.

"Would you like some squash?" I asked Michael and our friend Kevin, who was helping us with renovations.

"Sure," they said in unison, at which point I opened the oven door and squatted down to pull out the rack. It was then that I saw not one but two fat rats eating the warm, caramelized orange flesh of the squash.

"Oh, darling," I said to Michael, quickly shutting the oven door. "Would you like rat with your squash?"

"There's no rat there."

"Oh yes, there is. Right here, inside the oven."

Out of the corner of my eye, I saw the two rats scampering in single file along the far edge of the countertop. They were like soldiers on a reconnaissance mission, heading straight for the hole in the floor behind the fridge that would lead them to the basement and their freedom.

FINDING PINK

Karuna is the Sanskrit word for compassion. It is also the name of the yoga center where I was transformed from being afraid of becoming a mother to embracing the prospect more fully in my heart. Karuna is housed in an old Masonic temple adorned with gilded pillars and ornate moldings fit for the palace of Versailles. Practicing yoga in this luminous studio is like floating on a cloud; there is a lofty, heavenly feel to the room. It was in this sanctuary that I delved deeper than I ever had into the ancient science and healing powers of yoga.

When people ask me what yoga is, I often tell them it's like going to church, the gym, and therapy all at the same time. Yoga simultaneously strengthens and softens the body, that vessel we all inhabit that serves as a portal through which we comprehend and understand our experiences of the world. Through regular practice, traumas that have been lodged in tissues and organs and manifested as anxiety can begin to be released. Flexibility of the mind, body, and spirit flow easily and naturally as a result of yoga, leaving a practitioner with an overall sense of happiness and well-being.

Students who come to class expecting to "get into" poses quickly learn to honor and accept whatever their physical and mental state is on any given day. Yoga was my saving grace during fertility treatments; it helped me stay centered and sane. With the realization that my endocrine system might not fulfill its reproductive mission, my yoga practice gently reminded me to respect and honor my body—no matter what.

I was with my yoga teacher Eileen, my dear friend Leigh, and several other women at a retreat in Costa Rica the week I miscarried. Alarmed that I might experience medical complications in a developing country, my doctor had advised me to undergo a D&C before I left. He also wanted to conduct a fetal tissue analysis to ascertain what may have caused the miscarriage.

While the remnants of life seeped out of me that week, I woke at dawn each day to practice yoga with this small band of women. With the wisdom of a high priestess, Eileen guided us through deep meditations and *asanas*—the physical postures of yoga that have been passed from generation to generation for more than a thousand years. I will never forget lying down in the back of the room on day four just as the sun was casting an orange glow over the lush San Jose Valley. Eileen read us a Buddhist poem about walking in a desert and stumbling upon your own dead body, your own corpse, decaying in the sand. Birds and lizards are feeding off your flesh. You know you are still you, but just barely. In the next line of the poem, the wind has essentially sandblasted all your flesh away, leaving only your skeletal form lying on the earth. Then you see the sun blazing down, baking and bleaching your bones. Eventually your bones separate and scatter; the notion of the body as a body has morphed into disparate pieces, like a puzzle that once fit together. Form has been completely transmuted. Finally, the poem ends with your bones turning to dust, life recycling.

While Eileen read the poem, I was a complete wreck, curled into the fetal position in the back of the room, trying like mad to contain the wolf howls that my body so needed to release. At the end of class, we formed a small circle and checked in with each other to see how we were doing. I could not contain myself. I wept as I spoke about the way all of our lives were intertwining that week. Though I had just lost a potential son or daughter, Leigh was commemorating the eleventh anniversary of her daughter's death: Kate had died from carbon monoxide poisoning in an apartment in Brussels when she was twenty-eight, and Leigh still mourned for her every day. Yvonne had survived two bouts of breast cancer and was trading in a career in finance and restaurants to teach yoga. All of these women, except for me, had borne children. I felt blessed to be sitting among them, and yet I grieved for their losses; I mourned for their dead or wayward sons and daughters, and for offspring who had turned their backs on them.

Though the ironies and tragedies of life have never been lost on me intellectually, it was during this week in Costa Rica, among these mothers, that I began to *physically* decipher the universal experience of grief, loss, and fear from a strictly feminine perspective. Every one of us sat in meditation with some degree of fear in our hearts, but with confidence and love as well. At the same time we were grieving over the death of a child, we were smiling at the wonders of the rainforest. All emotions, all thoughts, all experiences were simultaneously and fleetingly experienced. Thoughts arise and fall away; the breath rises and falls away; a fetal heartbeat rises and falls away.

◆

Before I entered the Modern Age of Fertility, I was always drawn to the more masculine side of myself because, to me, that side symbolized power and freedom. To admit I was female was to admit defeat. Some women and men believe that having children is a way of wielding power in the world. You are everything to your children, after all. You are their environment, their moral post, and their ecosystem. A job well done is a happy, loving, well-adjusted child. Sadly for me, I still associated motherhood with my rather dreary childhood experiences. In my twenties and thirties, my emotional survival demanded that I avoid motherhood at all costs lest I find myself once again inside the hypocritical and dangerous jaws of nuclear family life.

Yoga eventually loosened the thick skin I had grown in response to my home environment and then later, in New York, to a city that became a convenient excuse to hide my vulnerabilities. I had to be efficient and fast and kind of tough to make it in Manhattan, so I called upon my Yang spirit to help protect and propel me. I paid little, if any, attention to my Yin, or female, side because I did not value it at the time. I viewed womanhood and femaleness as a liability that would prevent me from attaining the freedom that I craved more than anything else in the world.

I lived a fantastical macho-female-superhero comic-book life. I became a rugged individualist, refusing to retreat or cry out for help. I wanted to prove that I was strong and capable, and I went out of my way to show everyone I came into contact with that I could do anything I set out do. Unfortunately, in an effort to keep pace with my boyfriend at the time, this included snorting too many lines of cocaine. One night I spent six hours in bed desperately gulping air while my heart pounded like a herd of angry elephants. I thought I was going to die.

My personal quest to prove I was bulletproof also meant traveling alone to Africa, where I came so close to being beyond stupid in my judgments that I am lucky the State Department did not have to intervene.

"Why are you going to Africa by yourself, for God's sake?" my father asked me as I packed my clothes and my only weapon—a Swiss Army knife—into my backpack.

"Because I can," I answered, swaggering like a tough guy as I loaded my luggage in the car.

The truth is that, during this pinnacle and life-changing journey to Africa, I was at times very lonely and frightened. I was scared the night I naively allowed a Muslim man I barely knew named Mohammed Ali to lead me through the center of town—four paces behind him, mind you—to his family's mansion on the island of Lamu off the coast of Kenya. When the tide rolled in and blocked my departure, I knew I'd made a terrible mistake. I stayed awake all night wondering if he would molest me and then kicked myself a thousand times for thinking that I might be the one Western woman who could educate him about equality between the sexes.

I was anxious again a few years earlier when, traveling alone in Paris, I succumbed to the advances of a Romanian graduate student I had met on the street. In his attic apartment he shared his desire to make love to me all night long—and safely—with a condom because "HIV and AIDS was very bad in Eastern Europe." When I decided I didn't really want to be in his bed, I ran blindly out of the building into the strange dark avenues wondering why I had given a stranger who reeked of tobacco, lime, and body odor permission to stick his tongue down my throat. The truth is, I did all these things and more because I wanted to prove that I could make life decisions based on desire and not fear. I wanted to prove that my safety—and my femaleness—didn't matter, even though I knew they did.

❖

Moving to the country with the purpose of creating a family and living a more balanced life initiated the unfastening of the armor I had worn for so long. Much to my horror, the more yoga I did the softer and pinker I became. I started wearing lipstick and bras again. I began to experiment with the notion of living my life without filtering every encounter through a political and gender lens. I wondered if it was possible to exist as a woman—a human being—without the weight of cultural propaganda and the truths about womanhood pushing in on me and coloring my experience.

At first, I was *terrified* to walk alone in the woods, not only because of my fear of getting lost but because I had grown up in a culture that told women they should be afraid when they walked alone in the woods.

Though I desperately wanted to be Daniel Boone, my victim-trained mind always filled with thoughts of renegade mountain men hiding out in the hills and hunting me down. As my yoga practice deepened, I became more adept at separating these mental fears from the physical reality around me. Yes, there was always a chance that a crazy man might sneak up behind me but that could happen anywhere, in my own home or on the streets, as well as in the woods. The truth is that, walking in the forest, I was far more likely to run into a deer or a porcupine scrounging for grubs in a rotted log. The more illuminated the inner workings of my mind and its effects on my body became, the more often I laughed at and drew connections between them. Slowly but surely, I started going for more walks by myself in the woods. Slowly but surely, the habitual pit in the stomach I had first acquired in childhood began to slough off. I became calmer, which allowed me more emotional and intellectual freedom. Perhaps, for the very first time in my life, I was finally beginning to feel the relaxation and spacious sense of openness that comes with being well loved and safe.

❖

By the time I turned forty, my career had become the center of my life and my purpose for living. It was the identity by which I measured my value and my worth. Many of the high-powered women I worked with did not have children. These feisty Baby Boomers were my mentors and my role models. They seemed happy. They had cash in the bank and black town cars with chauffeurs who drove them wherever they needed to go. They were female VIPs convening with heads of state, speaking at conferences, changing the world, I thought, for the better. When I was in my twenties and thirties, I wanted what they had.

Once Michael and I were married, he often tried to discuss with me the difference between *having* a career and *being* my career. In my case, there was little room for separation; I cared too deeply about the health, environmental, and social justice issues I worked on. Though he tried many times, it was nearly impossible to pull me away from research I might be doing on female genital mutilation or the number of malnourished children in India. Once, he came into my office while I was putting finishing touches to a 100-page policy report. He just stood quietly for several minutes while I ignored him, and then he said, "Babe. You've been at the computer for eight hours. Come on, it's time to stop."

"No, I can't," I said, tapping away at my keyboard. "Not right now. I have a few more pages to go."

"That's what you said an hour ago. Come on. You haven't even left your desk to pee."

And then he did the unspeakable. He placed his right index finger on the "Off" button on my computer keyboard. I went berserk.

"How *dare* you shut off my computer?" I bellowed. "This report is extremely important. The way I craft the arguments in this report could mean the difference between donors providing funding for a fifty-million-dollar literacy project for women and girls or a twenty-million-dollar project. The more money, the more women reached. If women could read, they could have better jobs, they could protect their children…"

Michael looked at me without saying a word and then left the room, closing the door behind him. Alone in my office, I realized that I had once again made the universal suffering of the planet more important than my own life—perhaps even my marriage. Michael helped open a tiny crack in my heart that day, which eventually led me to the visceral recognition that my career, while valuable for a whole host of reasons, wasn't the only thing in life that mattered. The trouble was the more I'd let go of work as my primary sense of self, the more vulnerable I felt. For two decades, my identity had revolved around my trying to save the world by influencing policy and public opinion. Who was I if I wasn't doing that?

A day came, of course, when this illusion about the life I was trying to control and manifest finally did begin to crumble. It was the moment when I actually heard the quiet voice buried deep inside me that I had been ignoring for a long, long time.

After several logistically challenging years slogging through our commuter marriage, I began to feel the first pangs of motherhood. I was very careful to submerge these sensations, placing them far out of view behind all the other "important" deadlines I needed to meet. Despite Michael's gushing endorsement of my kindness and compassion, I was still terrified that I would fail as a mother. I would lose control not a few times but most of the time. I would play mind games. I would have trouble negotiating my primary love for Michael with my love for my children. I didn't want to be inside what I still considered the dangerous circle of family dynamics again. Once was enough. At the time, the only solution available to me was to avoid the subject altogether. I knew this wasn't fair to Michael, but I had no choice. My deeper healing and exorcism from my past had not yet occurred.

One weekend, we went to a creativity retreat in upstate New York. It was the kind of retreat where as an adult you play with finger paints, make a kite and fly it, and, despite your lack of musical talent, join a band. The organizers invited every participant to submit a biography that would be turned into a booklet and shared with the whole group.

Most sent in profiles that read something like this:

> Hi everyone. My name is Rita. I am a recently divorced mother of three. My life is very difficult right now, and I thought this creativity retreat might inspire me and bring me more joy.

Another one read:

> My name is Henry. I love golden retrievers and chocolate ice cream. I used to be an artist before I sold insurance. I want to see if I still love art as much as I did as a kid.

Mine read:

> Miriam Zoll is an author and researcher for the United Nations. From 1990 to 1999 she served as a consultant to domestic and international public policy institutions focusing on women's reproductive health, HIV/AIDS, and human rights...

You get the picture. I didn't know what flavor ice cream I liked anymore and I couldn't begin to tell you if I was happy or sad. I saw myself in a whole new light after I read that little blue booklet. I began to notice how, at parties, I often spoke about my work but not about my personal life, or my non-work-related dreams. I realized how guarded I was. When had it become so hard for me to let my human vulnerabilities show? Had I become so used to defending myself from the potential landmines of office politics that I no longer knew how to genuinely relate to people?

The answer was yes. I had done what millions of Americans do in order to compete in a workforce as competitive as ours. I had transformed into the professional labels I had acquired because I thought I might lose my edge if I didn't. If I lost my edge, then I might lose everything else I had worked so hard to accumulate—my reputation, my status, my income, my referrals, my illusions about myself. Without even knowing it, I had morphed into what I was either rewarded for accomplishing professionally, or thought I should aspire to if I wanted to make it to the next level. That weekend, I somehow found the courage to admit that I really wasn't cut out for the petty antics of office politics. I disdained meetings where the ego-driven players of the institutional hierarchy threw darts at each other across polished cherry conference tables. I realized that I no longer wanted to be one of those women being driven around in a black town car and rushing off to the airport. What I needed to do was dig myself out and rediscover what was important to me.

I didn't even know if I still enjoyed my work, most of which had been focused on helping women and girls acquire greater political and economic power—no surprise, given my family background. Having witnessed up close what appeared to me to be my mother's un-empowered life, I realized at a very young age that choice and economic independence were the most important liberties for all individuals, but especially for women.

When at the age of seven my friend Diana told me her parents were getting divorced, I secretly wished that my parents would, too. That way we wouldn't have to listen to my father yell at my brother every day and maybe we wouldn't have to go to Hebrew school, either. As an adult woman trying to understand the complexities of my own love relationships, I asked my mother why she didn't leave my father when he became so impossible to live with.

"Where was I going to go, and how would I have taken care of you kids?" was her only reply.

In a world of fast-tracked, college-educated women, my mother's high-school diploma was worthless, and she knew it. Enduring the bumps and bruises of her marriage was the only choice she thought she could make. I was at least relieved to know that she had contemplated leaving, that she had at least thought it was necessary to protect her children from harm.

Shortly after that creativity weekend full of epiphanies, Michael and I rented a sailboat in the Caribbean. One night, I slept directly below the open deck hatch of the front cabin staring up at a fat white moon. It was on the boat that I gave myself permission to daydream about creating a life that might actually be balanced and rich. What would it be like if I switched careers, or had a child, or did both? If I switched careers, what would I do? How would I earn money? One of my greatest talents was mapping out and implementing new strategies to move individuals and organizations toward their goals, but, when it came to my life and my goals, I kept coming up empty-handed. There were no quick fixes anymore, no easy-to-access entry or exit strategies. I had to simmer uncomfortably in this No-Man's-Land-of-Limbo-and-Despair, otherwise known as encroaching Middle Age.

To ease my mental anguish, I began making a list of ideas that ranged from living aboard a marine research vessel from Woods Hole Oceanographic Institute to riding my bike through New Mexico to opening a yoga studio in a small coastal town. Soon that list grew to thirty items, which I then pared down to ten, and finally to four: sailing, yoga, dogs, and having a baby—in that order. While a baby still wasn't at the top of my list, I had at least been able to curb enough of my old resistance to have it make the final cut.

ADRIFT

After Costa Rica, still unable to accept our infertile state, Michael and I met with a younger fertility doctor who we thought would be more up to date than our other doctor about the latest hormone cocktails and reproductive technology innovations. He lost no time telling us that a female baby is born with millions of egg follicles that dwindle to about 400,000 when she reaches puberty. By the time she is my age, what remains are the eggs that were never very healthy to begin with.

"The strong ones leave the roost early," he explained. "The robust eggs want to move out. They want to meet the sperm. The weaker ones stay behind."

"Of course," he continued, unable to resist the temptation of his clinic's mantra, "that's not to say that you don't have some good eggs left." Ah, there it was: that glistening shiny hook, that single ray of hope that maybe this doctor could give us something the other couldn't. He also shared with us the results from the lab's fetal tissue analysis. The fetus I had miscarried had been male and chromosome pair #14 had been deformed.

"It's a blessing it aborted," he told us softly. "It's nature's way of selecting survival of the fittest." Michael and I said nothing, our thoughts locked on the knowledge that, had that pregnancy lasted, we would have had a son.

"After examining your charts, the way I see it, you have four options. You can live a life without children. You can try another IVF cycle with a new drug that is known to be highly effective. Or you can try a donor egg or adoption."

Michael and I had already been living a life without children. We had enjoyed many adventures together and we loved each other deeply, but when all was said and done we did want to have a family, which was why we were going through this hell in the first place. At this time, option number one no longer seemed like an option to us.

"We'd like to try again," we said in unison. We had talked about it before the meeting, truly believing that if we had been pregnant once we could surely do it again, and this next time it would work.

"Okay then," he said. "We need to wait one month for your cycle to normalize and then we'll start up again."

Another month? I hated hearing those words. At this point, another month equaled another year to me. Time was moving very quickly during this arduous process. Each menstrual cycle meant the loss of more eggs that could potentially become a life. Each month meant I was thirty days older. I complained to Michael that I did not want to be fifty years old when I delivered a child.

"You won't be, you'll be forty-three," he said. To me, that carried the same weight as fifty.

❖

We began our fourth IVF cycle with new super drugs in April. This time, Michael and I took turns with the injections. Just as it had one cycle earlier, injecting myself gave me that comforting illusion of power and control over my own destiny at a time when I desperately needed to feel that I was in the driver's seat. After ten days of shots, suppositories, and vitamins, I went for my first ultrasound appointment. As usual, the room was dark when I hopped up on the table and put my feet in the stirrups. I had never worked with this particular technician before. She was a bit more talkative than the others had been. I told her that this was my first cycle since the miscarriage.

"Well, let's see what's happening in there," she said with a smile, as she greased the probe and slid it into my vagina. She pushed first on the right side and then the left, measuring here and there, making tapping noises with her fingers on the keyboard.

"Okay. That's it."

"That was fast," I said, as I stood up.

"There's nothing there," she said. "The doctor will call you."

Did the technician really say there was nothing there? I was still bleeding every month, on time, regularly, like I've done since I was 11 years old. My blood was still a rich red, not some sickly brownish color. I was healthy. I was strong. But it simply didn't matter. No matter how clever I thought my arguments were, the doctors' tests and Mother Nature kept proving me wrong. Even with this hyper-egg-stimulating hormone, my ovaries were too tired to run the race. It seemed as though I was now more infertile and pre-menopausal than ever before.

Michael was deeply perplexed by the news.

"How can you have eggs and become pregnant one month and then only two months later have none at all?"

With great humility, we both recognized that human innovation could push the biological envelope only so far, and that ultimately it is still Mother Nature who decides. We found ourselves at a new impasse. If these drugs had been our only hope to spawn a biological child, we now had only three options left to consider: a donor egg, adoption, or life with no kids.

Our doctor gently reminded us again and again that, despite my shortage of fresh, healthy eggs, I was in fine physical condition to carry a child to term.

"Women four or five years older than you are giving birth to healthy children with donor eggs," he said. "I'm fairly confident that you could too. You're still young."

I was thrilled to learn that as a possible donor egg recipient the clinic would reclassify me as "young" instead of "old." It was too bad that I now considered myself to be almost too over the hill to even keep trying. Maybe it was okay for some women to give birth when they were forty-eight or fifty, but it wasn't okay with me; something about it didn't feel right. I had read the news article about a New Jersey woman who birthed twins at the age of sixty, and about Rajo Devi, an Indian woman who supposedly birthed a baby girl at the age of seventy! Were these medical victories over nature really something to celebrate? As Ann Patchett captures so vividly in *State of Wonder*, her novel about the desire for eternal fertility, aging, and the onset of menopause and conditions like osteoporosis significantly alter women's strength and endurance over time. Pregnancy at those ages poses serious health risks to women, not to mention the fetus they are carrying. Just because men who are in their sixties and seventies might continue to procreate (despite potential fetal health risks), it doesn't mean that women in the same age group can, or should. As for me, I could end up with 22-year-old eggs, but I would still be a middle-aged woman wondering how on earth I was going to muster the energy to be a first-time mother in my forties—the same age my friend Leigh was when she became a granny.

◆

We learned that the donor egg industry was earning thirty-eight million dollars annually and growing by 6 to 8 percent each year. A 2007 *New York Times* article reported that out of 15,175 donor egg cycles performed every year in the United States, 5,449—roughly only one-third—resulted in live births. Our clinic staff optimistically shared with us their belief that a woman in her forties had a 50 to 52 percent higher chance of conceiving using eggs donated by a woman younger than thirty. To average laypeople like us, these sound like great odds. But, as we found out months later, most women in their forties have a only a 1 to 2 percent chance of conceiving with their own eggs—which means donor eggs may increase their chances by only 2 to 5 percent. A friend of ours in California who is also in her forties confirmed this for us. During an informational meeting with her fertility specialist, she was told that her chances of conceiving with a donor egg were only 4 to 6 percent—hardly the numbers our clinic had shared with us. This misleading and mismatched bit of information made Michael and me wonder once again about how the industry and its clinics calculated their numbers and how we as consumers were expected to decipher and interpret them.

◆

"I just want to have a baby *now*," Michael said after the meeting. "I can't stand this waiting."

"I know," I said, giving him a big hug and a kiss. "I'm so sorry it's come to this."

Once again my feelings of guilt were crushing my insides. It was my fault we had a miscarriage. It was my fault my ovaries weren't producing. It was my fault we waited so long in the first place. I was a failure. If I had only tried harder to become pregnant we would have a baby now.

"Stop," Michael said to me. "Don't do this. You can't spend your whole life rerunning the what-ifs and should-haves. We both have regrets. Whatever happens, we'll be okay."

It didn't feel like anything would ever be okay again. Another year had gone by and we were still not pregnant. We were up against a wall we could not break through. All my life, I had been bold and precocious. As a kid, my nickname in the neighborhood had been "Boss of the Block," and even as an adult I was often called upon to help clients troubleshoot difficult situations. But how can you possibly troubleshoot a biological stalemate? I want eggs, and my body isn't producing any. How do you negotiate that with yourself? Up until this point, my life had always seemed so full of options and opportunities; it was just a question of tracking down the right information and the right contact person. But now, with my ovaries in retirement, I had no place to turn.

On top of all that, I really was losing my professional footing. No one pulled a switch and said, "Turn off Miriam's intellect and activate only her reproductive impulses." I did this all by myself as the process wore on, as all that poking and prodding below the hips began to dehumanize me. With so much of my time and energy focused on my gonads, I had slowly but surely neglected my brain and my career. The doctors and the nurses and the insurance agents did not care one iota about my work with African orphans or my research fellowship at MIT. The only thing that mattered was my hormones, my ovaries, and my pocketbook. Don't get me wrong. I am grateful that they cared so much about my organs of reproduction. That was their job. But I wonder what they thought about me the human being as I lay unconscious on the gurney. Did they feel sorry for my desperation, which kept them employed? Did they admire the fine structure of my ankles and feet while they were hooked into the stirrups? Did I have a face and a husband and a life, or was I just another older woman trying to have a kid?

❖

It seems fitting that during the summer of our miscarriage the engine on our sailboat suddenly conked out, leaving us adrift in the thick fogs of the Atlantic Ocean. On days when the winds did not blow we spent hours watching the flat surface of the sea while the sails flapped flaccidly from side to side. In those moments we wished and prayed for one good breeze, just as we had kept wishing for one good egg. Eventually the winds did pick up, but then the rain fell all summer long.

Figuring out whether to use donor eggs or not was a much more difficult decision for me to make than choosing IVF. There were many more ethical layers to wade through. For one thing, with IVF, I was the one making a conscious choice to try to make a baby by injecting drugs that could be harmful to my health. With donor eggs, I was asking a stranger to possibly risk her health on my behalf. That was a heavy burden to bear. The frustrating part of being caught in this web was that very little research had been conducted to determine if these fertility drugs were safe or not. No one knew. I was groping my way through this hellhole in the dark.

❖

Before fertility treatments, my annual interactions with the American medical establishment included one visit each to the dentist and the gynecologist. Once I turned forty, I added appointments for mammograms and for the dermatologist to check for skin cancer. Like many Americans, we paid thousands of dollars every quarter for our health insurance. Michael was the one who offered to wade through the bureaucratic muck to determine if insurance would cover IVF and donor eggs.

"You're sure?" I asked incredulously, imagining the hundreds of minutes he would have to spend on the phone on hold and the mountains of paperwork he would have to fill out.

"Yes, I'm sure. I'll worry about how we'll pay for this. You get pregnant."

As each cycle failed, we began to wonder if we were out of our middle-aged, middle-class minds to think that we had a chance of pulling this rabbit out of the hat. What I came to realize was that the insurance companies were thinking the same things. Unlike in countries where subsidized health care dramatically reduced patient medical fees, the average cost of one IVF cycle in the United States is approximately $12,500, and often more.

The deeper we waded into the reproductive technology process, the more complicated and expensive it became, and the more difficult it was to find coverage. Only fifteen states had laws mandating that insurance cover particular ART procedures—and only up until a certain age. With few, if any, insurance companies covering donor egg cycles, only the well-off or those people crazy enough to take out a second mortgage could afford the donor cycle fees, which on average cost $30,000.

These cycles could easily be compared to one of those very expensive adrenaline-rush adventure vacations favored by celebrities and the super-rich. They might, for example, pay a travel agency thousands of dollars for the privilege of skiing out of a helicopter hovering above a 20,000-foot mountain peak in Alaska. As they jump from the aircraft, there is always a chance that they might take the great leap and land on safe virgin powder with the perfect angle of their skis and have the thrill of their life. Or they might hit a rock face and die. Donor egg cycles are really no different. You are paying almost three times more than an IVF cycle for the *unlikely possibility* of becoming pregnant and *maybe* delivering a healthy child. It made no sense.

Before I had even begun IVF treatments, Blue Cross-Blue Shield had mandated that because of my age I would need to take what is referred to as the "Clomid Challenge." Clomid is often the first and least expensive fertility drug a couple comes in contact with. It is the drug that has spawned the birth of so many twins over the last two decades. In my case it was used to assess my ovarian reserve. If I failed the Clomid Challenge, Blue Cross-Blue Shield would not pay for any procedures related to fertility.

During the five days that I ingested this high-powered hormone drug, I became a raving lunatic. My mood swings were like that of a Category Five hurricane: one moment I was manically high and happy, the next moment in tears. It was a violent introduction to the world of fertility, but in the end I passed the test, and Blue Cross-Blue Shield agreed to pay for part of the treatments. We had subsidized the rest through MEGA Life Insurance out of Texas. Their local representative— a lean agent who with his leathery face and sinewy body was an easy shoe-in for the Marlboro Man—came to our house one day to make his pitch. As he was leaving, he gave me a pastoral look and offered some kind words. "Good luck to you," he said. "I hope this works out."

I was happy to receive his blessings, but I also noted the forlorn tone of his voice. During the months we relied on MEGA Life to pay, I kept wondering how on earth they stayed solvent insuring such risky medicine.

"Don't think about that," Michael warned me. "You'll jinx it."

After our fourth IVF cycle was aborted, we received a letter from MEGA Life informing us that our policy was canceled. From their point of view, it certainly made sense to pull the plug. Insurance companies want to pay for medical procedures with successful track records, which in the long run end up costing them less money. But the reproductive technologies we were trying were too unreliable and the success rates too low. MEGA Life disappeared at the same time as our last hopes of conceiving with my eggs did too.

❖

Sometime during this long, depressing process, Michael and I stopped making love as often as we used to. Apparently, we are not alone.

A 2010 Stanford University study published in the journal *Fertility and Sterility* found that infertile women were less happy with their sex lives than fertile women. Compared with the control group, the infertile group had significantly lower desire and arousal scores and a lower frequency of intercourse and masturbation. Before being diagnosed, however, they had enjoyed levels of sexual satisfaction similar to the women in the control group. Since fewer than half of the women had received IVF treatment, it was unclear whether or not hormone shots depressed their libidos, but the researchers believed the cause was mostly psychological.

Sex therapists like Ruth Markowitz in St. Paul, Minnesota, report seeing more and more couples whose relationships have been severely injured as a result of infertility treatments.

"The nonverbal message couples receive from everyone is this: do whatever it takes to have a child," she explained to me at a conference where we met. "And frankly, nothing else seems to matter, most certainly not your sexuality. Infertility is a problem directly related to folks' sexuality, so you can't *not* talk about it—though so few people do. So much shame comes in, anger, disappointment, and then to have to bypass those feelings and just have sex regardless of the emotions—it is enormously damaging."

By the time we reached the Donor Egg Dimension, Michael and I had both shut down, like robots whose battery packs were all used up. There was no juice left in the cells, no lights flickering on the circuit boards. Sex for us now meant stress. It meant needles and Petri dishes and stirrups. Sex was now associated with disappointment and guilt and pain. We needed Pavlov to come back from the dead to help reprogram us. We tried to reclaim and resurrect our sensual connection, but we just ended up lying on the bed like two beached whales gasping for air.

"I want to, but I don't know how anymore," I said.

"Me too. What are we supposed to do?"

We had no idea what post-IVF sex could be like, so we just lay naked under the sheets and held hands like a *New Yorker* cartoon from the 1970s.

"Do you think we'll ever have sex again?" I asked.

"Maybe," he'd say spooning me. "It doesn't work anyway. We failed to make a baby. Nothing matters anymore. We're at a dead end."

CAPITALIST CONCEPTION

I first entertained the possibility of working with a donor egg agency after the second IVF cycle failed. The very idea of Michael's sperm fertilizing *someone else's* eggs and then having those embryos inserted into my uterus made me wince. But, given what the doctors had told us about the quality of my eggs early on, I wanted to be open to the idea of a donor—just in case. While some of the literature said there was great success with older women using younger women's eggs, other data suggested just the opposite. Once again, it was a crapshoot: you either win or you lose, but the big question was, do you want to play the game?

The first donor egg website I happened to stumble upon was a California agency where the majority of potential donors looked like contestants for the Miss California pageant. They were all slender, blonde, and buxom and their price tags were high, ranging from $8,000 to $10,000. Why did they call them donors, I wondered? I spent only five minutes on the site before I hastily clicked off.

"There is no way in hell I'm going to put some stranger's eggs in my womb to make a baby," I told myself reassuringly. "We'll make a baby with *my* eggs."

I felt like an eggless sociopath for even considering asking one of these young women to risk her health so that I might *purchase* her eggs. The vast majority of donors on this site and elsewhere in the United States were in their twenties. How and why do they decide to sell their eggs to someone like me? How do the donor agencies and these young women determine that their eggs are worth $8,000 while someone else's eggs are worth only $5,000? Were blonde, blue-eyed donors always more expensive than brown-eyed, overweight donors? Were Caucasian eggs worth more than Asian, Asian worth more than African-American? We were told on more than one occasion that it is not unheard of for infertile Ivy League alums to post a classified ad in campus publications offering up to $100,000 for an egg donor with high SAT scores, 36-24-36 body measurements, and a penchant for Mozart.

Around the globe, the growing popularity of egg donation and its accompanying health risks and bioethical and marketplace conundrums appear to be lightning rods for controversy. Austria and Italy have banned donor eggs, and France forbids single women and lesbians to access ARTs in general. Canada banned the sale of eggs in 2004 but allows for altruistic donation, and Norway and Germany ban donor eggs but not sperm. In Sweden, couples must prove they have been in a stable relationship for at least one year before qualifying for fertility treatments, including donor eggs that are paid for by the state. Almost everywhere in Europe except in the Ukraine, couples are banned from hiring a woman to carry a pregnancy for them. Grappling with the ethical and moral questions the phenomenon raises, Italian law, most certainly influenced by the Vatican, limits the number of embryos created during an IVF cycle to three, and those must be implanted, not stored or donated. Australia, Brazil, Israel, and the United States impose the fewest restrictions on what is allowed in the marketplace.

In 2010 Arizona lawmakers did pass a bill that mandated unprecedented informed consent procedures to ensure that egg donors are aware of the emotional and physical health risks they may face. These include drug-treatment side effects, the depletion of their own egg reserves, and Ovarian Hyperstimulation Syndrome, a condition that can seriously damage a woman's reproductive system and, in some cases, even cause death. The year before, California legislators also passed a law requiring health risk warnings to be posted on all egg donation advertisements, but some say enforcement appears to be negligible.

Before our miscarriage, ethical discussions about the efficacy of donor eggs made for interesting dinner conversation, but now, faced with extreme circumstances, we began to reconsider what we had previously rejected. The more we talked about the possibility of using donor eggs the more anxious I became. In addition to our concerns about the donor's health, we knew that the vast majority of donor cycles did not result in live births. So why were we even trying? Did we still think we were special? Was I psychologically prepared to consciously invite someone I didn't know to implant her life force and genetic history into my body? Would I feel the same way if I needed a kidney or liver transplant?

As the donor egg debate consumed my consciousness, I dreamt one night that golden eggs were flying out of my uterus. This dream became a point of fantasy for me for several weeks. The would-be donor was transformed into a fairy godmother who waved a golden wand over my ovaries, making dozens of my own golden ova suddenly appear. The doctors preparing to extract them wore golden gloves and masks, and as my feet were hooked into golden stirrups they complimented me on the miraculous quality of my eggs.

"For sure, you will have a golden child," they said, flashing their gold-toothed smiles and Rolexes.

❖

The clinic required couples contemplating egg donation to attend one orientation meeting. The night we arrived, we were astonished to find the room full to capacity. Some couples were there because the woman carried a genetic disease, while others, like us, had tried multiple cycles that did not succeed. As I waited for the meeting to begin, I felt deep sorrow for everyone there. We were the majority: the patients who had attempted IVF but didn't go home with a baby in our arms. We were all shell-shocked fertility refugees who had been wandering through clinic corridors and operating rooms for months, if not years. We desperately needed comfort as we searched for one last lifeline before we abandoned the baby ship, yet that evening the clinic staff did not even offer us a cup of tea.

The social worker who led the meeting said nothing about the trauma and suffering that was so palpable in the room. She did not acknowledge our combined tragedies, the multiple miscarriages, the stillborn babies, and the millions of dollars we had collectively squandered on procedures that had not brought forth new life. Instead, she mechanically discussed the plain black-and-white facts about what an egg donor baby meant in terms of the law and insurance coverage. Once again, the clinic's cold and sterile approach—all business and no heart—made me feel neglected and mishandled.

"Depending on your age, some insurance companies will not cover donor egg fees," she explained to us. "Those of you with genetic diseases are more likely to be covered than those who have been diagnosed as infertile." She went on and on about the insurance policies and the state laws governing the rights of the recipient mother and father versus the egg donor. Finally, I raised my hand.

"So how exactly do we begin this process?" I asked. "As far as I know, we look through mug shots of young women who want us to choose them to be our donors, and we then make a decision based on who we think looks the most like the recipient mother?"

My question drew nervous laughter from the crowd.

"Yes, basically, that is exactly what you do."

The social worker explained that most egg donor agencies provide recipient parents with photographs and profiles of each donor they list on their websites. We learn a few things about the donor like her age, height, weight, and some self-reported family and medical history. Once couples select a donor, some clinics, like ours, but not all, require the recipients to pay for a series of rigorous tests to ensure that she is physically and psychologically fit for the job.

One couple announced that they had decided not to look at the photographs during their search for the perfect egg mother.

"We just want to know that the donor is a good person and that there is no family history of mental or physical illness."

Everyone in the room stared at them. The social worker was silent for a moment and then said something like, "Yes, it is true. There are some couples that don't care what the donor looks like."

That's a noble thought, but the idea of paying $30,000 for a donor cycle and *not* knowing what the egg donor looked like was akin to buying a piece of high-priced artwork unseen. I suppose some high rollers had the guts to do such a thing. I did not. It was difficult enough to accept the fact that *none* of my genetics would be passed on to the child. I wanted to know as much as I could about the donor, inside and out, and if possible, I wanted her to look at least a little bit like me. Michael felt the same way. If he was going to mingle his sperm with an anonymous ovum to create a child, then he wanted to see what he was buying, too. Though we were both extremely uncomfortable about selecting a donor and genetic traits for our offspring, we also felt there was something to be said here about consumer rights. Regardless of how the language of "donated" eggs was framed in the legal context in the United States, we painstakingly acknowledged that we might in fact decide to purchase another human being's genetic material, ancestral history, and appearance. That was a lot to swallow.

Slowly, people started asking more questions.

"Can a donor donate more than once?" one man asked.

"Yes, she can," the social worker answered. "Many times a donor will help a couple become pregnant, and then they will work with her again if they decide they want to have more children."

Michael asked a follow-up question.

"It is possible that we might have a successful pregnancy using a donor that someone else in this room has also used," he said. "If that happened, then our children would be related through the egg donor, and that means that everyone in this room has the potential to be related to each other. Is that right?"

There were more nervous murmurs as all eyes fixed on the social worker. We were moving into very dicey territory about the composition of modern families created through the use of technology and the new ethical concerns it presented. Sperm banks and fertility clinics were not keeping track of how many children were being born from donor technology. There were no restrictions on how many times or at how many facilities men or women might donate their gametes. Apart from the Donor Sibling Registry that helps donor-conceived children locate their half-brothers and -sisters, there was no national registry to track, share, or update vital medical and genetic information so essential to children's well-being and to public health. I watched as the social worker took a deep breath. She obviously wanted to be careful about what she said next.

All she said was: "Yes, that is correct. One donor could supply eggs for multiple couples in this room."

A bunch of us let out a little laugh, and then someone mentioned a story in the *New York Times* about a sperm donor who spawned an offspring pool of 150 sons and daughters, many of whom are in touch with each other in person or through the Internet. This led to another discussion about whether an egg donor has the right to meet a child conceived with her ovum.

"The recipient parents decide if they want their donor to meet the child," the social worker explained. "Sometimes couples want their children to have that opportunity and sometimes they don't. In many cases, once you sign the legal agreement with your donor, she will want nothing to do with you or the child once it is born. She wants to be anonymous."

A few minutes later, the program nurse walked in, and the topic turned to the medical rather than the sociological aspects of conceiving a child with donor eggs. During this segment of the meeting, we were told that one of the reasons why an egg donor costs so much more than a sperm donor is because of the health risks involved.

"A dedicated egg donor makes a huge commitment to the recipient parents," the nurse explained. "She commits to going through a series of rigorous psychological and medical screenings. If she is approved, the donor must then adhere to a very structured medication schedule.

She is basically going through an IVF cycle with extremely potent drugs and potentially harmful side effects. In some cases donors have produced up to three dozen eggs in one cycle."

"Three dozen?" several of us sitting around the table exclaimed at once.

"But a woman only produces one egg per menstrual cycle," Michael said. "By taking these drugs she will be depleting her own reserve and lessening her own chances of having children."

"Yes, that may well be true," the nurse explained, "but it's her choice. The drugs stimulate hyper egg production so that recipient parents have a supply of quality eggs that can be fertilized and some embryos that can be frozen for future use. If the first cycle fails, you can then use the frozen supply without having to ask the donor to begin again from scratch."

When the meeting adjourned, Michael and I looked at each other.

"What do you think?" I asked him.

He just sat there and shrugged his shoulders. He didn't know what to say. Neither did I.

❖

One thing this boom in fertility medicine has done is to help us apply an economic value to women's reproductive labor. This may or may not be a good thing, depending on how you look at it. In today's U.S. marketplace, an egg donation is valued at anywhere between $5,000 to $100,000 or more, depending on her bloodline. On average, though, let's say an egg donation is worth between $5,000 and $10,000. Some people think it is immoral to put a price tag on genetic material and women's reproductive hardware and capabilities. But, considering that the global fertility industry generates billions of dollars a year, why not calculate women's potential economic earnings, too? Surrogates in the United States, at least, are usually paid anywhere between $75,000 and $200,000 to carry another couple's pregnancy to term. Why not apply the marketplace values generated by surrogates and egg donors to healthy women who have conceived on their own? A typical mother of four, for example, would be compensated $20,000 immediately— $5,000 per egg—simply for the use of her eggs. Then, since she is carrying the fetus to term, she would be paid an average of $100,000 per pregnancy on top of the initial egg fee. That would roughly translate into a total of $420,000 just for those four reproductive cycles alone.

That same value is calculated at a lot less in Eastern Europe and in India and other South Asian countries, the fastest growing region of the "reproductive tourism" industry, a new niche of the global medical tourism phenomenon. More and more poor women are crossing borders to sell their eggs and rent their wombs to childless couples from wealthier nations, primarily the United States and Europe. In India, for example, where the Indian Council of Medical Research regulates fees, women earn a fraction of the U.S. rates—anywhere between $2,000 and $10,000 for surrogacy and between $250 and $400 (all USD) for eggs. Some consider this exploitation; others say it gives women a chance to earn unprecedented wages that can drastically improve their family's well-being. Is the West colonizing poor women's bodies, expanding their employment opportunities, or both? Having spent much of my time at the United Nations researching new global initiatives to combat female poverty, this sure feels like a strange remedy to me.

❖

Many sleepless nights later, and with much trepidation, we decided to move forward with a donor egg cycle. It was extremely difficult for me to accept the notion that I might become a birth mother to a child that would have no genetic connection to me. I was at once grateful for the technological options available to us and at the same time confounded that these choices even existed at all. It seemed at times like an inhuman choice to have to make, and one that we would not even be considering if we didn't have the resources to pay for it.

We signed up with a reputable donor egg agency recommended by our clinic. It required a $5,000 finder's fee up front, in addition to the $5,000 or more we agreed to pay a donor after her eggs were harvested. Once we signed the formal agreement and received our password, we glued ourselves to the agency's website—the electronic umbilical cord that linked us to the possibility of sparking new life.

There is a local diner near us that serves Blue Plate Specials on certain days of the week. Fridays, they offer fish and chips or a fried scallop plate. Saturdays, they make pot roast or turkey with stuffing and gravy. Thursdays were Blue Plate Special Days at the donor agency because that was the day they posted new faces on their website. Unlike the California agency I had glanced at a year earlier, this website did not feature Barbie dolls for sale. The faces that appeared on the screen were much more varied. Most of them were white Christians or Catholics who said they were donating so that all couples could experience the joys of parenthood. There were only a few Jewish donors, and even fewer Asian, Hispanic, and African American donors. Though some requested that homosexual or non-Christian couples not have access to their eggs, the vast majority of these young women didn't care who received their eggs. That first week Michael and I initiated our website search together.

"This is really weird," he said as we scanned through the photographs and files and squirmed with discomfort. "It's like hunting for something to buy on eBay."

We learned a lot about ourselves while searching for the "perfect" donor. We were astounded at how quickly we judged others based on their appearance. We both found ourselves saying things like: *This one's eyes are too close together. I don't like her teeth. She looks bi-polar. She looks uneducated.* This isn't necessarily a bad thing. Like any protective parent, you want to be discriminating when choosing the genetic code and physical traits of someone whose egg will form half the DNA structure of your potential offspring. But most days we were sadly disappointed that we found no one we felt "connected" to. As the weeks wore on, we developed our own particular editing style.

Since mental health was a really important criterion for both of us, the first thing we did was browse through the entire inventory of donors to see who appeared to be emotionally stable and who did not. This process usually removed about 40 percent of the available donors. Of the remaining possible contenders, we spent a longer time looking to see if any of them actually resembled me. That usually eliminated another 30 percent from the pool. We were left with women who might look a *little* bit like me, and who we thought, from first glance, were fairly stable in mind and body. From that point on, we would read through their profiles.

This was actually very time-consuming detective work. Twenty pages long on average, the profiles included information about the health and ethnicity of the donor and her family. If we didn't read carefully, we could miss the fact that a donor's grandmother had diabetes that later blinded her or that a donor's father had died of cancer. These were important details that could influence the health of the child later in life. Only a handful of women had taken the time to provide in-depth background about their personal lives and their reasons for donating. While most mentioned altruistic motivations, Michael and I had read enough news reports to know that many had signed up so they could fund their education or buy a plane ticket to Spain.

I became particularly interested in a young mother with a bright smile who practiced yoga, thinking that she and I would have similar values. When I showed her photo and profile to Michael, he looked at me and said in a very quiet voice, "Okay." We e-mailed the agency and told them we wanted to put Donor #333 on "hold" and were told that we would be placed on a "waiting list." The agency's policy was that any couple could place a hold on a donor, but the couple that had been waiting the longest had priority over those just beginning their search. Since we were new, the agency informed us that we were the ninth couple in line for this particular donor.

"It is the only fair way to do this," the agency told us.

Fair? The truth was there was no such thing as fair anymore.

❖

It was around this time that I started going to the Smith College library to write this book, in part because I wanted to surround myself with the energy of fertile intellectual women. The doctors had told us that young women have about 400,000 egg follicles so I figured that, with an enrollment of 2,700 students, there were likely to be at least a billion follicles on campus. Perhaps some of that fertility would rub off on me.

There were days when I passed a young woman on the street and had to fight back the impulse to ask her if I might buy her eggs. It became a joke between Michael and me, one tinged with sadness and a certain element of abnormal social norms. Who on earth would walk through the streets of a city and think about removing eggs from someone else's body? Sadly, I would.

A SEASON OF INSOMNIA

In my efforts to eject myself from the constant ethical dilemmas I was having about using donor eggs, I suggested to Michael that he have an affair with an attractive woman and make some kind of arrangement to raise the child once it was born.

"It would be so much easier and more efficient," I told him. "There is no guarantee that I'll even bring a donor egg pregnancy to term. I'm old. We need a woman with a young body and young eggs."

The surreal experience of using donor eggs reeked of high-technology playing God. It reeked of my own narcissism and our *obsession* to procreate. Considering the millions of children already born who needed parents, was it really that big a deal that we birth a biologically linked child? While Michael remained undecided about adoption, I struggled with the shame I felt about being a "have," spending obscene amounts of money on extraneous medical procedures the "have-nots" could never afford. A study by University of Illinois professor Dr. Tarun Jain found that nearly half the patients at a large Massachusetts infertility clinic were Caucasian and had advanced degrees. More than 60 percent had an annual income of more than $100,000. Chinese and other Asian women were also overrepresented in accessing fertility treatments, while African-American and Hispanic women underutilized such services.

Since our miscarriage, I had become fixated on mortality and death, and during my chronic bout with insomnia this obsession escalated. For the first time, it suddenly dawned on me that I was possibly halfway through my own life. I became terrified that something awful might happen to Michael, that he might drive to the grocery store one day and die suddenly in a freak accident. When the phone rang after eight o'clock at night, I automatically assumed that one of our parents was in the hospital or had died. I read portions of Stephen Levine's brilliantly written book, *Who Dies? An Investigation of Conscious Living and Dying*, to better understand the cyclic nature of life and death in a Buddhist-Western framework.

With our hope to bear a biological child eradicated, it now felt as though everything was dying around me and inside of me. My hormonal system was dying, my red and white blood cells were dying, and my optimism in general was dying. I began to imagine what life would be like if all the people I cared about suddenly vanished, as I knew they one day would. The fear of death clung to my skin like a barnacle, grasping so tightly that I could barely breathe. In the early morning hours, I looked out the windows and marveled at how old the mountains and the stars were. How inconsequential we humans and all of our self-absorbed worries were in relationship to a mysterious universe that kept expanding beyond visceral human comprehension.

"What a flea I am," I told myself as I sank deeper into the quicksand of existential philosophy. I had studied enough yoga, Hinduism, and Buddhism to understand that we humans were as divine as the waterfalls and great mountains of the world. I did not necessarily think my human form was any better than that of a centipede or a dragonfly.

"There but for the grace of God go I," I would say while observing a snowflake on the windowpane.

From January clear through to the middle of April, I experienced chronic insomnia. Night after night, I woke at exactly four a.m. and wandered down to the living room at the other end of the house. There I would deposit myself on the couch or the floor and cry for hours into a pillow, being careful not to wake Michael. I cried bottomless belly cries that emanated from deep within my being. It was as if all the accumulated pain and grief of my entire life were now being set free, like a wild animal finally clawing its way out of a cage.

I cried for all the fear I held in my belly as a child and an adult. I cried for my father and my father-in-law's fear of death. I cried for my mother's encroaching blindness. I cried for my cousin who had died of a brain tumor at the age of eighteen. I cried for my sister, who had been so sick from cancer. I cried for the millions of Africans dying from HIV/AIDS and for the people of Iraq and Afghanistan who lived in fear of being killed by U.S. troops. I cried for the death of my dog, Luke. I cried for the death of my unborn child. I cried for Michael marrying someone else when he should have married me. And I cried for my brother, who during my season of insomnia went back to jail, this time for only six weeks, for vehicular violations.

◆

It had been my idea to organize a sibling reunion at Danny's house in central Florida. During the thirteen years he had lived there, Danny had invited me to visit many times, and I had always made some excuse. The real reason was that it was too painful to see him. It seemed to me that he was still living the adolescent, rock 'n' roll lifestyle he had lived before he was arrested in the '80s. He had a tough time keeping a steady job and paying his mortgage, and he didn't sustain relationships for very long. During the last decade, we had seen each other maybe six times and spoken on the phone only several times a year. I felt it was time to reconnect.

Danny greeted Rachel and me on his front stoop looking like Mr. Clean with bad teeth, tattoos, and body piercings. If he hadn't been my brother, I would have been a bit afraid to stand next to him; he had successfully cultivated an external veneer of toughness to protect his inner vulnerable self. That first night, he prepared a roast of beef from Wal-Mart and introduced us to his roommate, Bill, the son of drug addicts who had both served time in jail. When he was eleven, his father had given him half a gram of cocaine as a birthday present. Bill's mom was an *Easy Rider* magazine centerfold, not once but twice, before she became ill and obese. A recovering crystal-meth addict, Bill had moved to Florida from Denver, where he had built a reputation for himself as Billy Divine, the underground rave party DJ who felt the presence of God in his soul when he spun records and controlled the beat.

We also met Fred, who had spent ten years in federal prison for conspiring to bring a million dollars' worth of cocaine into the United States. Fred and his young girlfriend had two babies in tow: Neveah, Fred's niece, and Louie, his girlfriend's second child. Her first child was born when she was fifteen, and she said that, ever since then, she regretted that their father had custody of both children instead of her.

"I can't afford to keep my kids, but maybe one day I will," she told me. "Danny said you've been trying to have a baby and you can't. I don't have that problem. Guys just have to look at me and I get pregnant. Do you want to adopt?"

I wondered if she was thinking of placing Louie with an adoption agency.

"I don't know," I replied, staring her right in the eye.

"It's not that I am considering adoption for my children," she said cautiously. "I'm just wondering."

The other baby, Neveah—that's Heaven spelled backwards—was a bright, beautiful, curly-haired toddler who was born to a crystal-meth-addicted mother. For now, she and her two sisters were living with Fred's parents but it seemed that they would soon fall into Florida's foster care system. Sometimes Danny prepared meals for Fred's entire family because they didn't have enough money to buy both food *and* diapers.

"My mother just had an operation on her heart, so I quit my job to take care of her," Fred explained. "My dad is a retired truck driver, and we think he's going to have to have one of his legs amputated soon. We're still waiting to see the first of the state money we've been promised for taking care of the kids, but we haven't seen nothing yet."

When I asked him how the crystal-meth had affected the baby's development, he sadly shook his head and told me she was a spitfire prone to fits of rage.

"Sounds like a regular two-year-old to me," my sister said under her breath, but the doctors had told them that all three of the girls would likely be prone to substance abuse for the rest of their lives.

When I invited Neveah into my lap, she came eagerly and with a big smile.

"Maybe they are wrong about her," I thought. "Maybe I'm here right now because I'm supposed to find myself a child that needs a stable home."

For a few moments in my brother's run-down house, I thought he might actually be the Baby Fairy who would wrap a small bundle in linen and place it on my pillow. The truth was that Danny was the King of the Misfits, immersed in an outlaw world of ex-cons and people who were generally down on their luck. The highlight of our trip was going to Busch Gardens, where Rachel and I watched like patient parents as Danny and his friend Doug, both high on marijuana, rode every crazy roller coaster the tourist trap had to offer. Six times they went upside down in loops and twirls and spins, sometimes at sixty miles an hour, just so they could feel alive in the haze of their stoned state of mind. I know some people don't consider pot to be a serious addiction, but an addiction is an addiction as far as I'm concerned.

I once told Danny that I'd give him $10,000 if he'd flush his stash down the toilet. He laughed at me. "I don't have a drug problem, Miriam. I can stop whenever I want to."

"So stop right now then," I challenged him. "Never do it again."

Silence. He must have been thinking I was such a drip. Most of the people he knew used drugs. Just as religion had been the central theme of my father's life, drugs were the central theme of Danny's— and had been for a long time. I always thought he should have gone to school to become a pharmacist. He was an encyclopedia when it came to understanding how different prescription drugs affected the mind and body. He also knew which states were moving toward legalizing certain illegal drugs and which ones weren't. From his perspective, laws against mild drugs like marijuana were like Prohibition, and he predicted that one day they would all be legal. So who the hell was I to tell him to change his life? I sounded like a self-righteous sister of the Holy Anti-Drug Church. Who was I to say that numbing out your pain with drugs was any better than numbing it out with too much work or too much TV or too many failed IVF cycles? Who was I to pass judgment on him and his friends?

❖

The season of insomnia also marked the first time in my life that I stopped eating meat. I had tried many times to become a vegetarian but my carnivorous cravings always won out. Now I had no desire to consume the flesh of another living creature. There was something about a whole chicken in a pot on the stove that made me stop dead in my tracks. It felt like cannibalism to me. For four months, I ate only grains and vegetables and fruit. I grew more and more exhausted, and my already waning energy began to plummet.

Then one morning I woke up hungry for a visit to the gym. I instinctively knew I needed to jump-start my system again, and before the sun even rose I was out of bed and dressed.

"Where are you going in such a rush?" Michael asked from beneath the blankets.

"To the gym," I proclaimed. "I'm tired of being depressed. I'm going to work out, to feel my body again, to reshuffle the deck."

"You're manic," he said as he rolled over and went to sleep.

The machine I liked to work out on requires that you enter your weight and age to determine the best-suited routine for the day. I was unnerved when I punched the "age" button and the first number that jumped into the digital display was "20." It took only a few seconds to flash back to an image of myself in college swimming at a beach on the California coast. I had wanted to move there permanently so I could enjoy sunshine and fresh produce all year round, but I had been afraid to leave my family and the familiarity of the East Coast. When I brought my mind back to the gym, the mirrors across the way reminded me that I was now twenty-four years older.

"When did I become forty-four?" I asked myself. I felt so old. I felt washed up. But I rode that machine across a hilly terrain for an hour and finally did feel alive for the first time in months.

❖

As our decision to use a donor gained momentum, I lost my balance. I couldn't believe that I was consciously choosing to walk into this ring of fire. Under no duress, I was willingly signing my name on the dotted line. I was consciously manipulating nature for my own gains, my own selfish reasons. I wondered once again who I had become and what my values were.

For many weeks, my daily routines took on the color and texture of life viewed through the eyes of someone intoxicated with absinthe. The world around me began to resemble Toulouse Lautrec paintings, complete with exaggerated colors and shapes. In my mind's eye, seemingly harmless squirrels grew into disgusting rabid rats and strangers on the streets were not to be trusted. My world was becoming dark and sinister, but there was more to my dismay than skepticism about challenging Mother Nature. There was profound grief about losing my chance to contribute my gene pool to humanity.

I knew I was missing out on something divine, and yet through the promise of science I was being given the opportunity to experience some semblance of it. But for the umpteenth time in my life, I was once again standing on the outside looking in, observing but not participating in the process that was now going to take place between my husband's sperm and someone else's eggs. Was I out of my mind? I wanted someone to intervene, to give me a real glass of absinthe or lead me to an opium bar. I wanted something—anything—that would distort the reality we were intentionally creating and taking full responsibility for. Some kind of magnetic force—what my friend Meryl calls the animal instinct to parent—was urging us on. That force, Meryl told me, was the same force that the penguins exhibited in the much talked-about movie *The March of the Penguins.*

"Don't you remember what the penguins did in order to reproduce?" she asked me on the phone one day. "They endured sub-zero weather. They nearly drowned, froze, and starved to death. So you and Michael are wading through a vast terrain of reproductive technology, feeling like you've sold out to your love of nature. But you're no different from the penguins. You are treading where you need to tread in order to reproduce. You are walking through the blizzard, just like those penguins. It's just a blizzard of technology."

I wanted to hug her for comparing me to the penguins. They were so brave and determined to do whatever was necessary to lay and then protect their eggs.

"That makes me feel so much better," I told her. "I've been busy beating myself up for being narcissistic and using my class privilege to buy the technology necessary to make a baby."

"Why is your desire to have a child narcissistic?" she asked. "Your situation is no different from that of the seven billion other people on the planet. You are doing what all species do. You are trying everything possible to conceive a child."

"I am?" I asked in a small voice, grateful that she was reframing my internal debate.

"You are," she answered back. "Your maternal instinct is incredibly strong. Otherwise, you wouldn't be going through this hell."

Maybe she was right. Maybe this was simply a high-tech version of the penguins' Antarctic reproductive obstacle course. Maybe I was just another mammal making my way through the cold night in search of my young. I just had to jump through hoops most mothers never even knew existed.

Meryl made me realize that Michael and I possessed more courage to become parents than we gave ourselves credit for. Maybe we hadn't sold out to the medical establishment after all. We were trying to make a baby in whatever way possible and with whatever risks it required. It's the unnaturalness of this whole process that was so difficult to swallow. It smells fowl, like something rotting in the sun. It bespeaks my tired ovaries, my overcooked eggs. How could something so elemental and basic as conception become so complicated, so splintered, so laden with heavy emotion?

❖

One morning, I showed Michael a photograph of a young woman who had provided very detailed information in her online profile. Most of the other donors had responded cryptically to questions like "Why are you donating?" or "Have you ever been physically or psychologically abused?" This particular woman had gone to great lengths to communicate who she was and to explain why she had decided to donate her eggs. She talked about her family history, telling us that her parents had divorced when she was little and that her mother had suffered a nervous breakdown. The donor had been in therapy over the years and now had a strong and loving relationship with her stepmother. I was immediately drawn to her honesty and openness.

I clicked on her photo. "What do you think of her?" I asked Michael. On the screen he saw an attractive blonde with a heart-shaped face, young enough to be our daughter had we had children in our twenties.

"She has a nice smile like you do," he said. After he read through her profile, he turned to me. "I like her. I have a real sense of her."

"Shall I call the agency?"

"Let's wait a day. Let's think about it."

"Someone else might bid on her before we do," I replied.

He looked at me, feeling the pressure and knowing that I was right.

"Let's wait three hours and then decide."

"Okay," I said.

Of course I was watching the clock, and worrying about how Michael was feeling. Though he didn't speak of it too often, I knew this was a heavy burden for him. So many times over the years, he had told me that he wanted to see my face smiling back at him in the face of our child.

Half an hour before the close of business that day, he announced that we should go ahead and use this donor.

"You're sure?"

"Am I sure? How can you be sure of something like this? She *seems* okay. She seems nice, healthy. Honest. I like her honesty."

"Me too," I said, and then I e-mailed the agency.

They responded by telling us that we had three days to make a final decision. As far as they were concerned, Donor #888 was on hold in our name and if after seventy-two hours we still wanted her, she could be the one to supply us with eggs. As you can imagine, those were three very long days. We tossed and turned restlessly for two nights, curling into each other and wondering if we were doing the right thing.

"Are we making a mistake?" I asked.

"It is the only way," he answered back, a hint of surrender and sadness in his voice. "You will be the birth mother. Your blood, your amino acids, your spirit will be in the child."

"And half of it will be you." I smiled.

"Half of it will be me." I hugged him tight, pouring all my love into the skin of his back.

❖

We were having coffee at a local café when the final hour approached.

"We have to e-mail the agency in fifty minutes," I told Michael. If we did not adhere to that schedule, there was a chance that another couple could claim this young woman and we might lose our opportunity.

"Hmm," he said. I opened my computer and pulled up the photos of Donor #888. We stared at her face on the screen for the hundredth time.

"She seems nice," he said. "She's attractive. She doesn't look a thing like you but she is attractive."

"Sweet," I replied. We reread her profile. She liked theater and baking cookies for her colleagues at work.

"I'd do something like that," I told him optimistically. He smiled. A minute later a young woman walked into the café who could have been the twin of the donor whose face was now on our computer screen.

"Is that her?" Michael asked me.

"I don't know. It sure looks like her."

We studied the photo. Then we stared at the woman. "It might be her," he said. Finally after about ten minutes, the young woman asked if we could help her.

Embarrassed, we said, "You look like a friend's daughter. Are you from Connecticut?"

"Actually, I'm from California."

"Oh," we said, half relieved. "I guess you aren't her." But she could have been, and somehow that made us both feel okay about e-mailing the agency and telling them we wanted Donor #888.

❖

Several mornings later I woke up and told Michael I didn't think I could go through with the donor cycle. Tears were streaming down my face.

"I don't want to do it," I told him through sobs. "I feel like a monster."

He stroked my head. "You are not a monster. You are beautiful."

I looked back at him blankly, wondering how he could find the Medusa in his bed beautiful. I was a freak, an aberration of womanhood. It was my fault that he had to mate with a stranger in a Petri dish. It was my fault this young woman was going to risk her health for me. How could he embrace me when I thought I should be publicly flogged? All I could do was cry and cry and cry. I cried along with the heavy rains that fell all through the East Coast of the United States that April. I cried inches of tears, my face constantly stained, my nose stuffy with emotion. Part of me was afraid I would be judged by others as harshly as I was judging myself. I did not want to wear a scarlet letter that would show the world how I had failed as a woman to birth my *own* child. My glass was completely empty, my mind full of sadness, fear, and self-contempt. For two weeks, I did not sleep while the demons tossed and turned within me. Each night, I was visited by any and all thoughts that interrupted any chance for peace. I was in an all-out war with myself and my values.

❖

Once we chose Donor #888, we had to sign numerous documents outlining our legal agreement with her and with the clinic regarding embryo storage, donation, or disposal. Michael didn't react to the lawyer as negatively as I did, perhaps because he retained attorneys' services all the time for his business. But I was cautious. I had devoted a good portion of my adult life working to ensure that the courts did not interfere with women's and men's reproductive choices, but now I found myself in confusing new terrain: I wanted more protections in place to ensure the safety and welfare of families and their children, and for the egg donors and surrogates helping to build those families through reproductive technology.

My first concern was for the well-being of any potential donor-conceived offspring. There were few, if any, laws requiring clinics to keep their donors' medical records up to date. What if our donor provided eggs that resulted in sixteen half-brothers and -sisters and five of them developed a genetic disease? I would certainly want to know about it, but there was no national genetic registry where I might access that kind of information. With no mechanism in place to account for how many children are actually born from donor technology, there was also no public health authority tracking their health and development. This was disconcerting.

Having learned about the potential health risks many egg donors faced, I also wondered about safeguards for women like me who went through multiple IVF cycles. I tried not to think about cancer and other potential health problems that might arise from the potent hormone cocktails I had been consuming for the last three years. I didn't know if the risks I faced were less, the same, or greater than those facing egg donors.

Given the glaring absence of any long-term funded research studies tracking the health of women undergoing treatments, I did think that all clinics should be promoting the next best thing: the Infertility Family Research Registry. Housed at Dartmouth Hitchcock Medical Center, where its principal researcher is based, this voluntary registry has received funding support from the National Institutes of Health, the American Society for Reproductive Medicine (ASRM), and the Society for Assisted Reproductive Technology (SART). Its mission: "to learn as much as possible about the health and well-being of families built with the help of infertility treatment." To date, only seventy-six of close to 500 clinics in the United States have agreed to inform their patients of the registry's existence. Why haven't more signed up?

At the same time I felt the need for more protections, I also felt a very strong instinct to keep lawmakers as far away as possible from this most private matter. I didn't want the government, populated with so many elected officials who were ignorant about women's health and bodies and the struggles of infertile couples, to determine whether or not Michael's and my decisions were ethical or moral. Knowing that the egg donation would likely result in a number of healthy embryos remaining after transfer of one or two into my womb, we were now wrestling with difficult decisions pertaining to frozen embryo storage, donation, and disposal. We were now under pressure to determine for ourselves if we believed life began at conception or birth or somewhere in between. These were deeply personal and very difficult decisions to make, and we certainly didn't want state legislatures or Congress dictating to us when life began, or to prevent us from donating an embryo, or disposing of it, if that was our ultimate choice.

I knew that we needed to protect ourselves legally from ever having an egg donor claim a potential child as her own, which was why we were speaking to this lawyer in the first place. Still, I felt extremely anxious and mistrustful toward her. As with the medical staff, I didn't feel as though she actually cared about us—and most likely she didn't.

"You are making a business deal with the donor, and this legal agreement protects your interests and your investment," our lawyer told us over the phone with a thick South Boston accent. Of course she would think it was all as cut-and-dried as that; she hadn't spent the last four years picking herself up off the floor after failed treatments. I wanted to scream at her, but instead I bit my lip as she rattled on about the risks the donor faces. She told us that several weeks earlier an IVF clinic had retrieved fifty-six eggs from a donor using some new wonder drug. Michael and I were stunned. When we concluded the phone call, he turned to me and said: "This is an abomination. What are we doing?"

"Maybe we shouldn't do it," I answered, looking for a way out.

We sat quietly together for a few minutes, and then he confessed that, if the donor were a friend of ours, he would advise her not to go through with it. We were grateful that she was moving forward with us, but also frightened that she might hurt herself in the process.

❖

The very last question on the intended parents' questionnaire asked: Is there anything else you want the donor to know about yourself? I thought about that question for a couple of days before I wrote down my answer. I wanted the donor to understand that under ordinary circumstances I would never ask for her eggs. I wanted her to know that, given my entire life history and the circumstances of my birth, it had taken me a long time to realize that I could be a wise and loving mother. But now I was too old to embrace motherhood without sisterhood— her sisterhood, in the form of her eggs. Did she understand that we were making history together? Did she realize that at no other time in human civilization has a young woman had the opportunity to share her eggs with another woman so that she might become a mother?

❖

Though we chose our donor in February, the agency did not register our selection until they cashed our $5,000 check the following month. We then had to reschedule expired blood tests and wait another two weeks for the results. This brought us into April, when the doctor prescribed another round of birth control pills for me.

"It goes against all logic that when we're trying to get pregnant they put you on birth control," Michael said as I popped a purple pill in my mouth. I smiled but said not a word.

By early May, the clinic called to say that they were finally ready to administer the medical and psychological screenings, but they needed another $5,000 to start that process. We just bit the bullet and paid. I kept taking birth control pills, wondering if the transfer of the embryo would take place in July or August. We were both irritable, nervous wrecks. Maybe this wasn't the right thing to do. Maybe adoption would be better for all of us. Awake again at two in the morning, I questioned my ethics, or rather my lack of ethics. This tug-of-war went on and on, for each of us alone and for both of us as a couple.

Sometimes I sneaked downstairs late at night and looked at photos of the donor, convincing myself that she was a fine choice, that I was doing the right thing, and that she would be okay. I told myself that this was the twenty-first century, the modern age of science. Couples all over the world were employing technology to create families. In the back of my mind, however, I could never quiet that voice that told me I was being self-indulgent to a fault.

I asked myself in a whisper, "Does that mean that every couple in the world since Lucy"—that three-million-year-old *homo erectus* discovered in Africa—"was narcissistic for producing children?"

"Perhaps it does," I answered back.

"Does that mean that having children is always a compulsion?"

"Maybe," I said.

"Does that mean that little else in life matters except this animal instinct to reproduce?"

"Only when you reach a certain age, like you have. Only when the stable roots around you begin to decay and you know your own days are numbered."

"So," I said to myself, "you want a baby now because you know you're going to die. You think that having a child will make your acceptance of your own mortality less painful."

"Something like that, yes."

"That does sound selfish and self-absorbed, if I do say so myself."

"Yes, but maybe Lucy sensed her own mortality when she gave birth millions of years ago."

"Or maybe she just copulated with another hairy creature and didn't think twice about it."

◆

The clinic called a month before they were scheduled to harvest the donor's eggs and fertilize them with Michael's sperm.

"We can't allow you to use her eggs," said the nurse, who was in some ways beginning to resemble Nurse Ratched from *One Flew over the Cuckoo's Nest*. "She has a genetic disease that we just discovered as a result of the screenings. I shouldn't tell you this, but she is actually infertile. She will never have children herself, poor thing."

"Oh," I said numbly. "Poor thing."

"I'm really sorry," the nurse said. "I spoke to the donor agency, and they are waiting for your call."

"Thank you," I said robotically, wondering why this nurse offered no words of comfort about our devastation and disappointment.

It had taken me months to build a silent trust and relationship with this young woman, and now she was abandoning us through no fault of her own. She was oblivious to her medical condition, and state law does not require that donor egg agencies screen their donors for genetic disorders before they post them on their websites. It is standard procedure that recipient couples pay thousands of dollars worth of medical exams to ensure the donor they choose is fit for the job.

As consumers we felt that a $5000 finder's fee should ensure that the "product" we were buying would at least be fit for consumption. Perhaps Michael and I were the only couple who ever had the bad luck of choosing an infertile donor, but maybe it is more common than we think. To the agency's credit, they assured us that we would only pay the finder's fee once even it meant we had to choose more than one donor to find one that was appropriate for us.

After I hung up, I sat by the telephone for a minute or two just listening to the silence around me. "This is an omen," I thought. "This is a sign from the heavens that the path we have been walking is very wrong and that we should just accept Mother Nature's verdict and move on with our lives." Then I thought of Michael and how disappointed he would be if he went to his grave without ever having been a father. He will hate his life, I thought. He will hate me.

Michael was in the field behind the house with the tractor revving at full throttle. I kept waving at him but he did not see me. I screamed for him but he did not hear me. I screamed louder, tears clouding my eyes. Finally, he saw me, turned off the engine, and read the look on my face. Oh God, I thought to myself, he thinks his father has died.

"The clinic called," I quickly told him. "The donor we chose is infertile."

"Okay then," Michael declared with a hurt expression on his face as I climbed up on the tractor and hugged him. "This is an omen telling us that we should stop. Enough is enough."

Yes, I agreed, it was an omen and we should listen to its message. Then I started to cry and I told him no, it wasn't over. We could find another donor. We can't just give up.

When I went back into the house, I immediately pulled up the donor database we had spent so many of the last few months reviewing.

"Baby," he said when he came into the house a few minutes later and discovered me at the computer. "Don't do this now. We have to digest this news. Please don't stay on that website."

But I was obsessed, determined, and angry. "They made us wait five months. Five months and now we have nothing. I am going to be forty-five in three months. We don't have time to wait. We don't have time." I was hysterical.

He left me alone in my office with strangers' faces staring back at me. I found one woman who seemed "nice" and who was available for $6,000. I left her image on my screen.

"She looks nothing like you," Michael said when he saw the photo. "No way."

"The other one didn't look anything like me, either," I pleaded. "None of them look like me."

When I called the donor agency the next day, a new woman answered the phone. Our old contact was "out on leave," probably maternity leave, I thought.

"I am so sorry about your donor," she said.

"Me too," I said. "We never expected that a donor posted on your website would be infertile."

Silence.

"We were wondering what kind of priority status you are going to give us considering all that has happened. I assume that since we were one month out, we will have an opportunity to look at new donors before they pass onto the general website."

"Oh, of course, of course."

"Are we the only priority couple at this time, or are there other couples ahead of us?"

"Actually, there are three other couples in the same boat as you. For one reason or another, their donors fell through."

"So we might find someone we like and then whichever pathetic couple has been waiting the longest will have priority over the other high-priority couples? Is that how it works?"

"Yes, it does, but you are not all looking for the same traits in a donor."

I wanted to scratch this woman's eyes out. I wanted to make a Molotov cocktail and lob it through the front window of her office. Then I wanted to take a flame-thrower and drive to the clinic and burn the damn place down. I wanted to scream at the top of my lungs. I wanted to shove tables through windows. I wanted to yell at the nurse who back in October told us that the donor egg process had a much shorter timeframe than the IVF process. I wanted to tell them that they were all a bunch of liars who were selling false hopes to desperate couples who were regretting the decisions they had made over the last decade of their lives. I wanted to tell them that I was going to sue for fraud. I was going to sue them for making us believe that doctors and science and donors could make everything all right.

"No, I guess we don't all look alike, do we," I said sarcastically. "Well, do you have a picture of me?"

"No, I don't."

Of course you don't, I thought to myself. Why should you bother to see what I look like and who I am? I am the invisible, silent, pitiable woman who shells out money left and right so that you might pay your mortgage and monthly expenses. Why should I even think that you might have a photo of me on file? Stupid me.

"I'll send some right over."

"That would be great," she said, not suspecting my deep desire to craft a voodoo doll in her image so that I might stick it full of pins.

"By the way," she said, "did the nurse at the clinic tell you that a new donor came to us this morning?"

"No," I said, snarling on the other end of the phone line.

"I'll e-mail you her photo."

"Okay, great."

A few minutes later, the photo arrived. I was a bit baffled to find that the new donor looked enough like me to be a sister or a cousin. She had the same color eyes, the same cheekbones, and similar eyebrows and hair. She looked more like me than any previous donor in the database. Supposedly, this uncanny resemblance was the talk of the agency that day. The woman whom I had wanted to stick with voodoo pins was now my new best friend. I told her that I was excited but that Michael still needed to review the photos and her profile.

"Take your time," she said. "We'll put this woman on hold for you until we hear back."

We were very optimistic when we learned that this mystery woman had helped another couple become pregnant a few months earlier. Though we didn't know if the pregnancy had resulted in a live birth, we did know that this donor had a child of her own. Everything about her seemed perfect until we discovered that her father had multiple sclerosis.

"Forget it," Michael said immediately. "How could they even offer her to us as a donor? Her father has a serious disease. There is a chance that, if we have a child with her eggs, then our child might get this disease, too. We would live our whole life wondering when MS would strike."

"The agency is calling the clinic to ask the doctor what he thinks," I said.

"I don't care what the doctor thinks. I know what I think. This is a huge risk and I don't think I want to take it."

"*But she looks like me,*" I pleaded. "It's freak fate that the day after we lose our first donor this other one turns up and she looks like me."

"She doesn't look like you," he said. "She has the same eyebrows and eye color, but that's about it."

"But that's more than any of the other faces on this screen," I said to him, pointing at the mug shots before me. "Let's at least wait and see what the doctor says about the MS."

A few minutes later the phone rang. It was Michael's mother telling us that my father-in-law was in the hospital again. "It's nothing," she said. "Some fluid build-up in the lungs. Nothing too serious but I wanted you to know."

Tick-tock-tick-tock-tick-tock.

An hour later, the same nurse who had informed us about our first donor's infertility called to tell us that the clinic doctor believed it would be fine to move ahead with the second donor.

"He says that MS is very random in terms of who gets it," she said in her cheery, saleswoman voice. "It should be fine."

I thought this was great news. It meant that we would be able to finish the egg transfer before my birthday, which was important to me. Michael wasn't as elated at the news.

"Of course they say it's fine," he said angrily. "They don't want us to wait, either. I'm not so sure about this. It doesn't feel right."

"I know, I know," I said. "But the doctors at the other clinic thought it was fine to use her, and she succeeded in getting a couple pregnant in February."

"But we don't know if that resulted in a live birth."

"True, but she has her own child. She is under the age of thirty. She looks like me."

We thought it over for twenty-four hours, researching all we could find on the Internet about multiple sclerosis. Everything we read confirmed what the doctor had said, that MS strikes very randomly, that offspring may not be more susceptible to it than non-family members. After talking to a few close friends, we decided to move forward with Donor #2. I felt a deep relief that we were staying on schedule, that I would become pregnant before my forty-fifth birthday.

THE WAITING GAME

The waiting time in between cycles and tests and procedures is probably the most challenging period of the fertility process. For every day that I was not fully engaged with injections or ultrasounds or paperwork, I had time to question what we were doing and why we were doing it. I had time to look at myself in the mirror and wonder if the child would look more like Michael or more like the donor, or like the donor's great-great-grandfather.

The *New York Times* magazine published an article about children born through egg donation and the shame recipient parents say they experience as they decide whether or not to disclose the truth about how their family came into existence. The parents say they hesitate out of fear that their child might be ostracized or suffer other forms of social stigma. I wondered if the parents of children conceived with donated sperm felt that same heavy weight on their shoulders. As I read the article, I contemplated the notion of shame and stigma. Why was it that we humans experience shame in the first place? Did it erupt when necessary as some kind of internal monitoring mechanism, or was it only detectable when we believed outsiders were looking in with their hearts full of judgment?

The human condition seems to dictate that we all brandish a scarlet letter in one form or another at some point in our lives. It may be caused by an old embarrassment, dating back to elementary school when you stole a handful of hard candies at the penny store. Or it might be a much greater indignity like the one I carried about Danny's status as an ex-con. I hated those dinner parties where the conversation suddenly turned to discussions of prison reforms or prisoners themselves. At those moments, my face would heat up, and the old fight-or-flight response would surge in my belly. "Please, someone change the subject," I'd pray silently to myself as the dialogue droned on.

One time at a party a woman I had just met turned to me and said, "Can you even imagine knowing someone who has been in prison?"

I didn't respond, knowing that, because I was a white middle-class woman like her, she had simply assumed that I would never come in contact with someone locked up behind bars. Like me so many years ago, she thought "other" kinds of Americans—the poor, the broken, and the non-white of skin—wasted away in cages behind the thick walls of our nation's penal institutions.

I remember the first time I went by myself to visit Danny in prison. I was twenty-two years old and I felt incredibly out of place. The visitors in the waiting room were mostly women and children of diverse ethnicities and ages. There were heavy-set Hispanic women wearing leggings, high heels, and bright lipsticks, and withered Asian grand-mothers with small children in tow who had ridden the bus since early morning so they might steal a few precious minutes with their wayward sons. The young African-American and white women wearing push-up bras and tight jeans seemed to feel at ease and knew exactly what to say when the guards asked them a question. Then there was me, sitting there nervously waiting for my name to be called.

I kept telling myself I was nothing like these *other* women, repeating over and over in my mind like a mantra, "*I'm not like them. I'm not like them. I'm not like them.*" My sociology textbooks, the media, and American culture had taught me that poor people and bad people went to jail. Brown- and black- and yellow-skinned people went to jail. But if that was true then how did *my* brother end up behind bars? Nothing seemed to make sense anymore. The world no longer worked the way I thought it did. By my fifth visit, humility had settled on me like a soft blanket. The boundary of otherness that had been so pronounced on previous visits had vanished. I now realized that I was just like these other women, and that my brother was just like the other men locked up in the cells next to his. Any sense of advantage I thought I might have possessed based on my skin color or income bracket suddenly faded from view. I was no dif-ferent, no better and no worse, than anyone else in that prison.

❖

Michael and I quickly decided in favor of open disclosure with regard to the egg donation. On the advice of some friends and the clinic staff, we had been quite secretive about our fertility treatment experience so far. The clinic had advised us not to talk about it because "people wouldn't understand." But once we decided to share our decision about using an egg donor everyone rallied to our support, which we desperately needed.

I had overcome some of the feelings of inadequacy that I felt when we first started wrestling with the decision to use a donor, but I still felt deep sadness about it. Michael couldn't understand why I was so upset. He was troubled by it, too, he said, but it was just a donor egg. Just a donor egg? If we were using donor sperm, I wondered if he would feel the same way. I ventured to guess that, of the many couples that attempt to make a baby with donor eggs, the women more than the men have at one point or another felt some sense of shame about their decision and about themselves. I was willing to bet that women judged themselves more harshly and negatively than did their male partners.

◈

When I was a little girl, my sister and I had identical dolls that slept in identical bassinets. The only difference between them was their hair color; Rachel's doll had blonde hair like her and mine had brown like mine. We played mommy to those dolls every day for years, changing their diapers, feeding them with bottles, nursing them through imagined sicknesses. Though we weren't aware of it, we, like billions of little girls around the world, were being groomed for motherhood.

The assumption that all women will one day become mothers is ingrained in every culture and every religion. There is no question that for many women biology drives the desire to bear offspring. But what about the ones who aren't driven by biology at all? What about the women who have children because their priest told them to, or because someone once called them abnormal for not feeling maternal? How do these forceful external social and cultural pressures play out in the psyches of women who are ambivalent or afraid, as I was, about having children?

A childless older woman is still regarded in many circles as a pariah. In India and some countries in Africa and Latin America, a barren woman is marked for life—and sometimes literally branded or scarred by acid—and often treated with disrespect. I remember, during one of my trips to southern Africa, meeting a group of women in a village near Lake Malawi. They were washing clothes and bathing their children at the water's edge when I came along in my two-piece bathing suit, with a batik scarf wrapped around me like a skirt.

They were laughing as I approached.

"Hello," I said to them smiling.

"Hello," they answered back in unison as their children turned away from their water games to stare at me.

"Why are you laughing? What is so funny?"

The women giggled and pointed to my exposed belly.

"Where are you from?" one of them asked.

"I am from America. New York City."

Screams of delight and then, "How many years are you?"

"I'm thirty-two."

"And how many children do you have?"

"Me? I have no children."

They looked at each other, the wrinkles on their brows growing deeper like the ripples in a pond. It was unfathomable to them that a woman in her thirties was childless. In their country, women my age were already dead from the HIV virus, or if they were still living many were already grandmothers. I was an aberration in their eyes. I wondered what they would have thought of my plans to birth a donor-egg baby.

❖

One day, well into the waiting game with Donor #2, I received a phone call from the nurse. She told me that the clinic couldn't move forward with the donor's medical or psychological screenings until Michael and I contacted the financial office.

"Why do we need to call finance?" I asked. "I believe we are all paid up."

"You have to pay for this donor's screenings," she said.

"But we already did. We paid $4,000."

"That actually covered the first donor," she replied. "You have to pay for each donor's screening."

"Are you telling me that we have to pay $4,000 again?" I was livid.

"Well, yes, of course," the nurse said matter-of-factly.

"But that's ridiculous. The second donor just completed a cycle at a reputable hospital clinic that resulted in a pregnancy. Why can't you use their tests?"

"Well, we have to run our own tests. All tests must be conducted within the last six months."

"Her tests should still be viable. I think you should check and see if you can use their data."

"All right," she said reluctantly, realizing that I was not going to give up the fight. "But you have to realize that we have to make money somehow. These tests can't be free."

"You may remember that our first donor was infertile. She had a genetic condition. It doesn't seem right that we should have to pay the full four thousand again."

"Let me see what I can do. I'll talk to the doctors and get back to you."

I hung up the phone, shaking with rage. Michael had been talking about the money lust of the industry for many months now, but I had wanted to believe that they actually cared about us. I didn't want to get angry with the people who were trying to help us start a family, but this last interaction put me over the top.

This nurse was the same one who had told twenty exhausted fertility patients that the donor egg procedures usually take about four months to complete once the donor was selected. We were now approaching the one-year mark and we still hadn't gone through a full-fledged cycle.

❖

While we waited for our donor's test results, it was hard not to think about all the couples who made love on some moon-drenched night and simply ended up pregnant. What a blessing that was, the old-fashioned way of making babies. No technological interventions or stopwatch intercourse. That was a luxury I could not even imagine any-more. I could only dwell on the relentless planning, the chilling sensation of the vaginal probe, and the vulnerability of the stirrups. There was no longer a whole me engaged in this process. There was just the shell of me going through the motions. Time and experience had taught me how to detach, and I now considered myself a full-fledged skeptic. I was now wary of all my interactions with the donor agency, because I didn't believe they had my best interests in mind. If so, they wouldn't have posted an infertile donor on their website. The clinics and the donor agencies had their payrolls and their profits in mind. After all, first and foremost they were businesses with bottom lines to meet and profit margins to hope for.

❖

In the end, the clinic did waive the test fee and the doctors gave a seal of approval to our new donor. I had spent most of the summer consum-ing various forms of estrogen and injecting myself with daily dosages of Lupron in order to ready my uterus. In the heat of July and August, on sailing trips and during dinner parties, I would discreetly saunter off in search of privacy so that I might poke my belly with the syringe. Two weeks prior to transfer, I went to the clinic for an ultrasound. They wanted to measure the thickness of my uterine lining. I passed with fly-ing colors. The minimum width they wanted to see was six centimeters. Mine was fluffing up at a nice six point six. We were ecstatic.

I told Michael I wanted to spend as much time on the ocean as possible, sailing and swimming. I wanted to escape from the trials and tribulations associated with being on land. I didn't want to think about the donor going under anesthesia for my sake. I didn't want to think about her little boy wondering why Mommy was injecting hormones again or how she earned $6,000 in six weeks. I didn't want to think about the clinic. I just wanted to float on my back knowing that my uterine lining was building up a soft cushion to protect our future progeny. I wanted to look up at the sky and smile at the sun and be grateful for science and all the bounty it was about to bring us. So we sailed and somehow, during these months of suspense, I found the fortitude I always needed to captain the boat by myself. I exiled Michael to the companionway and made him swear a vow of silence.

"If I need your instructions, I'll ask," I said, as I confidently stepped up to the helm. "Only speak if you think we're going to capsize."

I was still a fair-weather captain, to be sure, but that summer a new supply of courage surged through me. Michael looked at me with patient trepidation, attributing my bizarre behavior to the hormones.

I also became quite superstitious looking high and low for signs and omens that might confirm our impending pregnant life. One morning I woke up and saw a rabbit munching sweet grass in the yard outside the kitchen door. "Aha," I thought when I saw its furry tail. "That's a sign of fertility if I ever saw one." A few days later, there were more omens: a mother raccoon and her three babies, followed by a mother deer and her two fawns, and then a moose and a porcupine. My animal-loving friend Bonnie interpreted all these sightings to mean that I would have multiple births, and I had to agree with her. I also started speaking to my ancestors—the Jews and the Christians—for the first time in my life, calling upon them to lend their assistance, wherever they might be.

Several days before the scheduled egg retrieval, Nurse Ratched called to tell us the donor's ultrasound revealed that the follicles visible in her ovaries were large enough for retrieval. She instructed me to wear an estrogen patch that I changed every fourth morning as a complement to the two estrogen pills and the evening dose of Lupron that I was already taking.

On a Tuesday afternoon in August, Michael drove gallantly to the clinic to provide his sperm. That morning the doctors had retrieved a dozen of the donor's eggs, which the nurse said was a "very good number." We thought a dozen sounded like a lucky number, too. That was six more than my very first IVF cycle three years earlier, and twelve more than my last cycle. Double sixes are an exciting dice pair; there are twelve days of

Christmas, twelve months in a year, and Jesus had twelve disciples. The number twelve was a nice, round, even number. There was no question the odds were finally in our favor. By the end of the week, at least two healthy embryos would be inserted into my womb and lodge into the now ripe lining of my uterus. The remaining ten embryos would be frozen—along with 500,000 other embryos in deep freeze across America—in case we decided to have more children later.

Based on what I had read, medical technology could on occasion breathe life into an embryo that had been frozen for some time. I knew of a woman whose healthy five-year-old son had been timelessly suspended in frozen space for four years prior to his being implanted in his mother's womb. In cases such as these, I often wondered if the child was really five or was he nine? I supposed it depended on whether you believed life began at conception—whether in a Petri dish or not— or if it began when a child was actually born. These were the kinds of tough philosophical and ethical questions ART consumers were forced to contend with everyday but that most Americans did not necessarily even think about unless they were prompted by the media.

There was a disturbing article in the *Los Angeles Times* right before Christmas 2012 that described an anonymous donor embryo program at a clinic in Davis, California. For the last couple of years, California Conceptions had been uniting anonymous donor sperm and eggs in a Petri dish and selling the resulting embryos in the marketplace—three tries for $12,500—a "bargain" said Ernest Zeringue, the clinic doctor who initiated the program. Those that aren't sold to patients are considered clinic property and stored in an embryo bank.

This was not the first time a clinic in the United States had offered such a service to its clientele. In 1997 the *New York Times* reported that Columbia-Presbyterian and Reproductive Biology Associates were offering "ready-made embryos." A New York State court later ruled that embryos were to be created only at the behest of patients, not for the purpose of storage in an embryo bank. In a similar case in 2007, the Texas-based Abraham Center of Life's embryo program was initially investigated by the FDA for operating out of the founders' house and purchasing eggs and sperm from "attractive" donors at wholesale prices in order to make "designer babies." The FDA later ruled that the case fell out of their jurisdiction, but the center did eventually close down.

Like these other clinics, California Conceptions believed that their program reduced a couple's costs and the length of time they might have to wait to receive a donated embryo. The clinic claimed that success rates were high, with some pregnancies resulting in twins. There were happy families out there, to be sure, but a much bigger question needed to be asked: Did we really want to be selling potential human life in the marketplace? It's one thing when a couple donates their frozen embryos to another family, but to actively engineer an embryo with the specific intention of selling it?

That is another question all together, and one that the American Society for Reproductive Medicine's (ASRM) ethics committee was scheduled to debate in January 2013. In truth, it really doesn't matter what the ethics committee decides. They don't have the power to enforce standards and protocols, only to suggest them. California Conceptions' donor embryo program made me think of the assembly line at the Ford Motor Company factory in Detroit. Do we really want to go there?

◆

While we waited to find out how many of the donor's eggs had been fertilized with my beloved husband's sperm, the nurse instructed Michael to administer progesterone via injections into my buttocks, alternating cheeks each day. These intramuscular injections were delivered via a thin two-inch needle that forced a thick solution of progesterone and sesame oil into my body. After my first dose, my buttocks were so sore I could barely walk. I was almost in tears as I told Michael that I didn't know how I could possibly withstand these shots for six weeks, in conjunction with the roller-coaster suspense of waiting to find out if we were pregnant. We had just begun researching the possibility of substituting a progesterone suppository for the needle when the phone rang. It was the doctor's office.

"What have you been told about yesterday's retrieval?" our doctor asked, once we had both picked up a phone.

"Just that you were able to retrieve a dozen eggs and that they were fertilized with Michael's sperm," I said.

"Yes, that's right. But I'm sorry to say that I don't have good news for you. None of the eggs were fertilized. I'm sorry."

I was speechless. Of course the doctor did not have good news for us. The clinic never had good news for us. Only once in four years did we receive good news, and that turned into tragedy with our miscarriage seven weeks later. Rather than fighting back tears, I now found myself fighting back an insane urge to giggle. All of our efforts to conceive now felt like a never-ending Monty Python skit. Laughing seemed to be the only way I could cope with this newest slap in the face, but I kept my lips sealed and let Michael do the talking.

"But there were twelve eggs. None of them fertilized?" he asked softly.

"It's really quite shocking to us," the doctor said in that tone of voice we had heard before. It was the tone that implied the clinic was not responsible for this outcome—and I suppose in many ways they weren't. Doctors could try to manipulate nature, but they could not control it completely. From their point of view, we had chosen a donor, they had approved her as a candidate, and done the best they could with the eggs she had produced—supposedly. Secretly I wondered if they had dropped the eggs on the floor, or if perhaps the thermostat in the laboratory was not set at the right temperature. There were a million possibilities for human error.

"I don't understand why this happened." Michael said quietly, absorbing the news. "Each time we did an IVF cycle with Miriam's eggs, they fertilized."

"Well, to be honest, we don't understand either," the doctor replied. "We've compared your sperm count from previous cycles to this one and they are comparable. There might be something wrong with your sperm that we haven't detected yet, and there is likely something wrong with the donor's eggs."

I didn't say a word. I just sat there listening, trying to make sense of all the reasons why the science had once again failed. Our donor had helped another couple become pregnant only a few months earlier. Maybe she should have taken more time off between cycles before working with us. Why hadn't the doctors flagged the possibility that her reproductive system was oversaturated with drugs that were likely wreaking havoc on her ovaries? Why hadn't we thought of that? But maybe the real reason this cycle failed was that Michael and I weren't supposed to have children. If we did have a child with this donor's egg, maybe it would have developed multiple sclerosis like its grandfather. Maybe it didn't work because Mother Nature didn't want it to. Maybe it didn't work because human beings weren't supposed to play God.

We had done everything we were supposed to do in this crapshoot except walk into the clinic's waiting room when I was twenty-five years old. We signed all the forms, wrote all the checks. I had filled myself full of hormones. Michael had ejaculated on command. It all boiled down to the fact that we had chosen two donors from a reputable agency, and in the end both were essentially infertile. One was twenty-one years old; the other was twenty-eight. And we, the desperate and hopeful couple, had absolutely no consumer protections. We had spent thousands of dollars on IVF and even more on the donor egg process and, through it all, the clinic was never held accountable for the outcomes. The pharmaceutical companies that made the drugs the donor and I ingested was not accountable. The donor egg agency was not accountable. The donor was not accountable. No one was accountable but us, really, because we were the ones who signaled everyone else to try to help us. And they did try. We could have chosen ten more donors and perhaps none of their eggs would have resulted in a baby, either.

While I half listened to Michael's conversation with the doctor, I had an epiphany that actually made me smile. I realized that for the first time in five years I didn't feel responsible for this particular failed conception. I had absolutely nothing to do with it. I was just sitting on the sidelines.

"I do hope you will try another donor cycle, but I don't recommend you use this woman again," the doctor advised. "Though she did produce a pregnancy for another couple, there is obviously something not quite right. Given the drugs she was taking, she should have produced many more eggs than she did."

Once again, I held my tongue. Thousands of dollars earlier this same doctor had told us that Donor #2 was a fine candidate. Apart from her father's multiple sclerosis, they couldn't find anything wrong with her. Now he was recommending that we not use her again. Instead, he was encouraging us to spend more money and select a different donor, perhaps a younger donor or a donor with purple eyes and blue hair, who might give us a better yield. What kind of wishy-washy medicine was this? Was I punishing the clinic for not living up to its end of the magical bargain, or did I have legitimate gripes? The more I thought about it, the more outraged I became. We had spent years following doctors' orders. We had rallied through the drugs, the heart palpitations, and the emotional roller coasters. We had willingly and under no duress paid ridiculous amounts of money for access to medical technologies that we were sure would work but never did. We paid for the chance to hope. We paid for the chance to try.

We are the only ones who are accountable.

NO ESCAPE

Within forty-eight hours of the doomsday phone call, we packed our bags and headed to the boat. I wanted no connection to land, no connection to other people. We were both somewhat elated to be at sea. We felt a sense of relief.

Michael confessed that he never truly embraced the idea of Donor #2 being the egg mother. He had not shared his reluctance with me during the weeks leading up to the retrieval because I was pushing so hard to stay on schedule and become pregnant before I turned forty-five.

"Her father has multiple sclerosis," he reminded me. "I kept worrying about that. Each morning I woke up and said to myself, 'It will be okay once the baby is born. It will have Miriam's blood in its body.'"

"Maybe your sperm knew that, deep down, you really didn't want to do it," I said softly. "Maybe you were being a protective father by willing conception not to occur."

He looked at me and smiled. It was so clear to us now that this second donor attempt, like the first, just wasn't meant to be. We could end the entire quest now, adopt, or keep trying with the technologies and drugs. It was still unclear what path we would choose.

Though we fled to the sea with the hopes of escaping, our fertility saga followed us like a lost dog in the night. One evening while we were having cocktails with Michael's thirty-something cousins Emma and Johanna, we started talking about the new egg-freezing technology the media was, in my opinion, endorsing too soon. While the potential impact of these $10,000 to $22,000 procedures *could* be as revolutionary for women under the age of thirty as the Pill had been, the technology was still too new to guarantee that every woman who tried it would birth healthy offspring down the road. Very few babies had been born as a result, and there were no studies assessing infant health over the long term. Nevertheless, the news sure was seductive.

"I wish I could have frozen my eggs when I was younger," I announced. "Imagine being forty-five or forty-eight or even fifty and still having access to your own thirty-year-old gene pool?"

"It'll never work," Michael said cynically. "More empty promises, more cash over the counter for the industry."

Emma and Johanna eyed us curiously and I think with a tinge of pity. When the waitress delivered my favorite summer drink—Bombay Sapphire and tonic with extra lime—an elegant, silver-haired man with a fine summer tan sauntered into the bar. He looked very familiar but I couldn't quite place him. Several minutes later, I realized it was the Silver Fox from the clinic, and my heart began to race.

I turned to Michael and whispered in his ear, "Is that the Silver Fox?"

He looked to where I was pointing, studied the man's profile and body, and nodded his head. Sure enough, standing before us was our very first fertility doctor, the one who had told us up front that I was too old to bear a biological child and that we should try donor eggs or adopt.

Michael whispered the newsflash to Emma and Johanna.

"As soon as we set foot in his office, he was the only one of the bunch who was truthful with us," he explained. "We just chose not to believe him."

"Not so," I corrected him, taking another gulp of my drink. "He gave us the bad news *but* then he reeled us in like all the others with that clinic mantra: '*It only takes one good egg.*'"

"Oh, right," said Michael chuckling. "He did say that."

"If he hadn't said it we would have walked right out, don't you think?"

"I'm not so sure about that. Who wouldn't wish on a shooting star? If they say it might work, then of course you try. You have no choice but to try."

❖

During our Great Escape, we both succumbed to the illusion that we had a new lease on life. We thought that with this chapter of our lives closing we could now put all our energy into figuring out what was next. I was oddly elated that I did not feel the guilt I usually did after a cycle failed. Michael was incredibly relieved that his sperm had not mated with an egg that might have carried multiple sclerosis into his offspring. Overall, the escapist strategy had lifted our spirits and made us feel hopeful for some semblance of happiness again.

But once we returned home, the crushing silence of the house and our derailed plans to turn a guest room into a nursery hit us hard. Insomnia crept back into my life, as did the remorse that had plagued me earlier. Looking at a baby picture of Michael one morning, I burst into tears, thinking that if he had never met me he might have grown up to become a father. He laughed out loud when I told him through tears that he should have married someone else.

"I did marry someone else, remember? It was horrible." He hugged me.

That morning I went to the eye doctor. The intake nurse reviewed my old records and noted that I had been pregnant the previous year.

"Oh, so I see that you were pregnant during your last visit but not today, so we can put those drops in your eyes and do some tests." I slumped in my chair a bit, my heart falling toward the floor. I didn't have the emotional strength to correct her. Five minutes later, she asked me how my one-year-old was.

"Actually, that pregnancy did not last," I told her softly. She was mortified at her faux pas and placed her hand over her mouth to admonish herself.

"I am so sorry," she said. "I shouldn't have assumed."

"It's okay," I told her. "Really."

She looked at me with the instinct of a healer and started telling me about an older woman she knew who had birthed a child with donor eggs. "Do you know about donor eggs?" she asked with a heart of gold.

"Oh, yes, I know all about donor eggs," and I told her how we had just tried a second donor and that none of the twelve eggs had fertilized.

"Not one?" she asked with wide eyes.

"Not one," I said.

"You must be exhausted," she said sympathetically.

"I am," I whispered back as tears welled up in my eyes.

"Would you ever adopt?"

"I'm not sure."

We chatted with this kind of openhearted intimacy for about half an hour before she had me read the eye chart. I could barely make out the letters and numbers.

"My eyes are getting old, too," I told her, "not just my eggs."

We both laughed as she ushered me into the doctor's examination room. He came in a moment later, this kind man who enables me to see the world. He too looked at my records and turned to me and said with a big smile, "Oh, so you're pregnant! Congratulations."

"Actually, I'm not. Those are old records."

"How old is your child?"

I died inside again. Was this really happening?

"Actually," I said, "that pregnancy did not last."

"I'm sorry."

I fought back tears as he looked deeply into my eyes with the help of those amazing machines that have fascinated me since I first started wearing glasses at age eleven. Could he see the sorrow permanently embedded in my retina? Did he see my forlorn soul? While he flipped through the various lens options, I was grateful for the kindness I found in this small country town where we lived. The staff I interacted with only once a year had inquired about my well-being and patted me on the back more than the employees at the clinic ever did during four years of treatments.

When the second doctor came in to examine my eyes, he too glanced at the computer file and saw that I had been pregnant during my last checkup.

"How's that baby of yours doing?" he asked with gusto.

Strange events come in threes, the saying goes, and so I braced myself for this déjà vu discussion. In a quiet voice, I told him that the pregnancy had not manifested. He immediately turned away from the computer, rolled his chair over to me, and looked me straight in the eye.

"I know that trying to get pregnant can be a very long and drawn-out process," he said sympathetically. "I have friends who have been trying for years. They went through so many ups and downs with treatments but they just came back from Montana with an infant in their arms. Adoption—you know? Instant baby."

Right, I thought to myself. As though that couple felt anything but "instant baby" in their long quest to start a family. The idea of slogging through the red-tape jungle of adoption laws and rules and regulations was overwhelming. We had just emerged from one swamp. Did we really want to get dragged through the mud again? Besides, we weren't sure we had completely given up on egg donation. If we were going to gauge our finances again, should it be for adoption or for the chance of having a half biological child? We had spent thousands of dollars on donor eggs without ever making it to the transfer stage. Were we crazy to think that it could actually work?

Several weeks later, Michael walked into my office and found me on the donor agency website again. "What are you doing?" he asked.

"I'm just checking out this month's available donors. You never know."

We started scrolling through the mug shots together as we had done so often before. This time, however, we argued about why one woman was acceptable while another one wasn't. Soon it escalated into a fight and then tears, and when Michael tried to console me I started pounding his back. Through a mixture of rage and sobs, I asked him how he could even consider asking me to go through the hell of the drugs and looking at these stranger's faces again. Why was he so wary of adoption? Once those words were spoken, I quieted down and we held each other for an hour.

These unresolved questions were torturous. In the dark hole of another sleepless night, I realized we were turning into caricatures of Edward Munch's famous painting *The Scream*. On this black-and-white canvas, a haunted figure holds his hands to his ears as he opens his mouth to scream, and the crazy, swirling energy of his inner world spirals around his head.

FERTILITY REFUGEES

There was a sign on the bulletin board in the building where I practiced yoga that advertised healing modalities to help women to conceive and deliver a child. Each time I walked by that sign I told myself to call, but I never did. I wasn't quite sure what it all meant but I was curious because the practitioner was also a *doula*, someone who assisted women during labor.

A month after the second donor egg debacle, I finally picked up the phone and dialed. I left a message for a woman named Susan explaining that we had been trying to conceive for five years. I knew that my odds were low but I was wondering if there was something she might suggest I do just in case we attempted a third donor cycle. When she returned my call, I told her about my chronic fight-or-flight responses, which had only grown worse over the last few months, and the racing heart that had plagued me off and on since I began hormone treatments. I also told her I was a bit frightened of delving into a deeper awareness of my body. Friends who had done this kind of somatic healing therapy had told me that it could be very powerful and some-times overwhelming as the physical body began to release old traumas. I had been through a great deal over the last sixty months, and my body, and my heart, had taken the brunt of it. Did I really want to relive it all over again?

On a Thursday morning in September, I met with her for the first time. Within minutes, I learned that she was exploring the possibility of trying a donor egg cycle herself at a local fertility clinic.

"You're kidding," I said, slouching in my chair. "What are the odds of me choosing a healer who is also about to enter hell?"

"I debated whether I should tell you," she said with a smile, "but I thought it would be best if you knew."

"But what if my experience affects you in a negative way? I might feel like I have to censor what I say."

"Don't worry about that. I'm centered. Let's focus on you. What's happening?"

What was happening? I felt like running out of the room, for one thing. I wasn't sure I wanted to sit there and tell someone I didn't know that my throat felt permanently choked and that my heart kept pumping faster than a racehorse. I couldn't pull myself together, that's what was happening. I was a wreck. But rather than spilling my guts all at once I started by telling her that I had trouble breathing.

"I can't seem to inhale any breath into my abdomen. It gets stuck in my throat and my chest. I'm suffering from insomnia again and I have constant anxiety in my belly."

There. I confessed. I told this complete stranger that my body and mind were twisted like a pretzel and shut down, and that one of the most basic of bodily functions—filling and deflating the lungs—was not functioning properly.

"If you have a constant pit in your stomach, it makes sense that you can't take a deep breath," she said. "Your muscles are working overtime and gripping. Let's see if we can begin by having you sit upright in the chair. I notice that you are quite hunched over and collapsed."

Quite hunched over and collapsed? She was being polite. I *was* the Hunchback of Notre Dame; I was the letter "C." I looked like and had the lethargic energy level of a ninety-year-old woman burdened by the emotional weight of so many years of life.

"Can you sit up straight in your chair? Just put your back against the chair and lift your chest. Close your eyes and let your hands relax."

My back creaked as I tried to sit up straight, and when I took a deep breath, I sensed it descending a millimeter lower than it usually did.

"Good," she said excitedly, observing my posture. "Did you feel that?"

I nodded my head yes as tears welled up in my eyes.

"She noticed my existence," I thought to myself with glee. "She is my witness. She sees that I have been drowning, and she is throwing me a lifeline. Bless her."

After a few more minutes of slow, deep breathing, she helped me lie down on the massage table.

"Give your body time to sink down and relax," she advised. "Close your eyes and place your hands on your belly. Take a deep breath through your mouth and draw breath down, down, down into your belly. Fill your womb with breath. Fill the ovaries."

These were hard instructions to hear. She was going right for my fertility-trauma jugular, but I did as she asked for several minutes before she invited me to make a sound on my next exhalation.

"Whatever sound is there. It doesn't matter what it is."

What emanated from my throat frightened me. It was a noise I had never made before. It was the mournful tone of widows crying in the deserts of Arabia—the woeful sounds of death.

"Another deep breath into the belly," she said, coaching me to go deeper and deeper each time while she drew my chin to my chest and lengthened the back of my neck to release tension and free up my nervous system. On the twentieth breath, my body unleashed a torrent of tears. The sobbing came from some place deep inside me. It was my body's turn to grieve now, for the needles, the stirrups, the sedation, the miscarriage, the vaginal probes, the ultrasounds, the blood work, the hormone injections, the pills, and the dashed hopes. I cried in her office for an hour and continued crying for three days, knowing it was only the beginning. The phone rang on the third day. It was Susan.

"How are you doing?" she asked cheerfully. "I wanted to check in with you."

"I'm okay, I guess. I've been crying nonstop. Is that what happens? I come in, I talk a little, and then I cry for the rest of my life?"

"No, not always, but often after the first session. Your nervous system is letting go of a lot of stored grief and energy. It's okay. You'll be fine. Just be gentle with yourself."

I went to a second session two weeks later and then canceled the third. I was terrified of my emotions and my body. The work we did together was helping to dissolve the pit in my stomach, but it was very taxing. An intense, burning fury was beginning to surface beneath my tears, and I didn't know what to do with it. My heart began racing again, just as it had during treatments. Often times, it felt as though a dozen Clydesdale horses were stampeding through my chest and I could not catch my breath. I knew it was my heart's way of telling me that, as dead and defeated as I may have felt, it was still there, alive and pumping. I forced myself to continue working with Susan because I sensed that new life could never root within my womb if it was competing for breathing space beside old traumas and demons.

Every dreaded session released another layer of fear and hurt that I had tried so hard, through talk therapy and yoga, to dissolve. I thought I had outsmarted my neuroses, but they had just burrowed deeper inside my body. Now I was freeing them like old ghosts let out of a long-locked closet. Lying there on Susan's table, I began to feel—perhaps for the first time in my life—that I was actually worthy of sympathy. I didn't have cancer, but I was affected by it when it struck my sister. A gun wasn't held to my head as I was handcuffed and sentenced to three years behind prison walls, but I was affected by it when it happened to my brother. Until now it had never been okay for me to grieve for myself. I had always grieved for others. That is what all these old tears were about: my failure to end other people's suffering and my own.

❖

I never thought I had much in common with Marilyn Monroe until I stumbled upon a YouTube documentary about her life. In 1962, after 20th Century Fox dismissed her from her final film, *Something's Got to Give*, Marilyn had a sinking feeling that her movie star days were numbered.

With thirty-two-year-old Elizabeth Taylor racking up forty-two-million-dollars' worth of over-budget fees during the filming of *Cleopatra*, Fox decided it no longer wanted to pay for Marilyn's hangovers or her tardiness on set. Incredibly astute at protecting her image and her career, thirty-six-year-old Marilyn reclaimed her waning sex symbol status by discarding the body suit she was instructed to wear for the nude pool scene. Instead, she gave Hollywood a fleeting glimpse of her bare self—a move that immediately resurrected her standing with studio executives and sold millions of fan magazines.

Despite her astounding abilities to seduce the public, Marilyn suffered throughout her life from severe depressions and insecurities linked to early childhood traumas, abuse, and years of living in foster care and orphanages. During her marriage to playwright Arthur Miller from 1956 to 1961, she lost two pregnancies. Unpublished clips from *Something's Got to Give*—shot just a year after her divorce from Miller—show a smiling Marilyn romping in the grass with the little boy and girl who play her children in the film. They are about the same age Marilyn's own children would have been had she not miscarried. According to her close friends, these interactions with the children compounded an already complex bipolar disorder and a tendency toward depression.

Since her death, America's mythmakers have linked her suicidal decline to her diminishing status as a sex symbol, her broken love life, and her addiction to pills. Rarely has anyone discussed how distressed she was over losing those babies and her chance to become a mother. Any woman who loses her ability to safely harbor new life—whether at seven weeks, six months, or thirty years—feels that loss with varying degrees of intensity until the day she dies. One might compare it to the universe losing its gravitational pull: suddenly everything spins out of control and planets and stars smash into each other. There is complete chaos and disorder, and life never quite reassembles again into that recognizable system of order. A chill would pass through me when I thought of the millions of women in the world who had lost children through miscarriage or violence or illness. I grieved for them as I grieved for myself, still, so many months after our one loss. I was again struck by the fact that, had our pregnancy flourished, Michael and I would have been holding in our arms a little boy composed of DNA from both of us. I didn't know how long I would grieve over this, or how long I would cling to it. I tried and tried to let go, but it kept creeping back inside my heart time and time again. When I gave it the attention it craved, I would have a good cry and then step back into the kitchen to pour myself another cup of tea. I was thankful for the daily rhythms and demands that pulled me back into the Game of Life, and I knew it was okay to move off to the sidelines every once in a while for another time-out. Unlike Marilyn, I didn't expect myself to smile for the camera every day.

Marilyn had been forced to contend with her loneliness and mood swings with barely any support from the outside world that supposedly adored her. Hollywood made millions of dollars from her fantastic hips and her ability to exploit for the studios what had been exploited in her. She could turn on that electric smile and that famous wiggle at the drop of a hat. But when the singing and dancing were over, when the cash at the ticket booths had been deposited in the banks, Marilyn returned to her bedroom alone. There she made love to her champagne and sleeping pills, seeking relief from that racing mind of hers. Looking for love in all the wrong places, she tried hard to be perfect and beautiful and talented so the studios and the public would never abandon her as her own mother had. But at the end of the day, they did turn their backs on her; 20th Century Fox's bottom line dictated that they discard her like an old gown in a wardrobe closet. Her loneliness terrified her. She was nothing without her acting, nothing without the studios, and nothing without her fan base. Was it any wonder that a woman so well-versed in turning into whatever the love object needed her to turn into would become the world's longest-lasting sex symbol?

❖

Just when the isolation of country living began to really wear on our nerves, Michael began a new building project in the Boston area. While he renovated the upstairs units in an old brick apartment building, we temporarily occupied the basement apartment. Most mornings, I was awakened by the sound of hammers and drills, and every once in a while plaster wafted down onto my head. Some days the dust and rubble were so thick he banished me from the premises.

As hard as it was living in the basement of a construction site, it was a necessary change. Every inch of the beautiful farmhouse we had worked so hard to turn into a home had begun to feel a bit like a shrine. We had moved there shortly after 9/11 to raise a family, and maybe some chickens and goats, too. Living there full-time after fertility treatments failed had simply become unbearable. The move back to the city immediately animated our energy levels. Michael was up at seven a.m. and didn't quit until six p.m., and the sounds of traffic and the subway made us feel like we were part of the human race again. Alone in the country, we had been mournful. Back in the city, we were simply one couple out of a million coping with life's losses.

Perhaps as a way of subconsciously punishing myself even more for not producing a child, I decided one day to have my hair cut. I didn't ask the hair stylist I had never met before to trim a couple of inches off my shoulder-length tresses; I asked him to make it very short—above my ears—so that I resembled a boy. Somewhere in the foggy bottom of my depression I had decided that amputating the symbol of my femininity might help sever my grief, too. When he was finished, I rose triumphantly from my seat like Wonder Woman and pumped my fist in the air.

"Good riddance to the past," I told myself, truly believing that without the weight of long hair on my head I might now be free to ascend to the heavens. While it may not have appeared logical to anyone else, that hair lying on the floor like a mound of dead snakes represented *all* the failures of the past few years. If cutting it off helped me rise up out of the depths of despair, so be it.

I was in the kitchen arranging a bouquet of flowers when Michael walked in to grab a glass of orange juice.

"Hi," I said. I flashed him a big smile and turned 180 degrees so he could view all of the New Me. He said not a word, just stared, and then went upstairs to the second floor and ripped down some more walls and banged a few nails.

"You don't like it, do you?" I asked him when he appeared a few minutes later covered in dust and wood chips. He looked a little dazed.

"I had no idea you were thinking of cutting your hair," he said, still staring at me to make sure I was the same woman he had been married to that morning.

"I didn't either."

"But why did you cut it?" he asked, slowly and almost hurt. "I loved your long hair."

"I cut it because it's time to turn over a new leaf," I replied with authority. "It's time for both of us to leave the past behind and start focusing on the future. I'm tired of looking like a hippie. Maybe if I have short hair I'll look more like a businesswoman and I'll be able to take the bull by the horns again."

"Oh," was all he said, as he turned around and walked out the door.

Three weeks later, of course, the fantasy that had propelled me to cut my hair in the first place wore off.

"I look like a boy," I cried to Michael one day. "Why did you let me cut my hair? You should have told me to just buy a wig."

"I had no idea you were going to cut your hair," Michael said, trying not to laugh as he soothed me.

"I am ugly and old and my hair will never grow back."

"Yes it will," he assured me. "Everything will grow back in time. But for now, I think you've done enough penitence. You don't have to drag yourself over the coals anymore."

Ha. That's what he thought. Little did he know that I had been methodically adding more salt to my wounds by obsessing over a bizarre reality TV show I had discovered by chance one night while channel surfing alone in the dark. I had been watching a program about a 600-pound woman who was recovering from gastric bypass surgery—she lost about 150 pounds in one month—and then clicked randomly to the Discovery Health Channel's "I Didn't Know I Was Pregnant."

The show featured reenactments of "true" stories about women from across the United States who had no idea they were pregnant until the moment they went into labor. Many of them never gained weight or missed their menstrual cycles. Some ended up giving birth during their own weddings or in fast-food restaurants or isolated campgrounds in the Pacific Northwest.

That first night, I just sat on the couch shaking my head in disbelief. I couldn't for the life of me comprehend how any woman could be pregnant and not know it. Perhaps they were just incredibly ignorant about their bodies. How could you not know you were pregnant until your water broke? When I told my friend Shelley about my latest masochistic compulsion, she laughed.

"Have you ever seen the program?" I asked her.

"No," she tried to answer in between giggles.

"These are supposedly true stories," I explained. "These women are living normal lives and then one day they feel intense pain and cramping and they go the bathroom only to find that the baby's head is crowning."

I heard more uncontrolled giggles on the other end of the phone.

"I know it sounds unbelievable," I told her, "but after an hour or so, these women emerge from the bathroom or the restaurant or the campground with a baby wrapped in a clean paper towel or a t-shirt."

Shelley still hadn't stopped laughing.

"Okay," I said. "Check it out and let me know what you think."

❖

One evening after Michael went to bed, I snuck onto the donor website again. There they were, those young women under the age of thirty-two. I clicked through each page, searching their faces frantically for clues about my future. Then I took a deep breath and realized that I was being manic.

"How many cycles do we go through thinking that maybe the next time it will work?" Michael had asked me after our second cycle failed three years earlier. "We could spend our whole lives trying to conceive."

We had in fact spent approximately 2,000 days trying, and here I was going right back for more. The donor's faces were like heroin now. The fertility treatments were like the needle. Our fixation with having a baby had turned into an addiction. But the truth was, I didn't feel desperate at that moment. That wasn't the right word. I felt something else, something I couldn't pinpoint. Part of what I felt was fear. Fear that I hadn't tried hard enough or willed it enough. Fear that if anything ever happened to Michael, then I would truly be alone in this world. Fear that when I died I would simply vanish from the face of the earth in a puff of smoke, like Merlin the Magician passing through time and space.

"Is this really it?" I asked myself.

Did living a fulfilling life mean that you had to have children? There were thousands of animal species that did not reproduce and millions of female homo sapiens throughout the ages who had been barren. In coyote culture, the alpha female has pups, and her sisters serve as supportive nannies, enabling the babies to mature under the watchful eyes of a whole community. Perhaps I was destined to be a sister and not a mother, and perhaps sisterhood could be as fulfilling as mother-hood but in a different way.

The more I thought about it, the more I realized I had already spent a great deal of my professional life as a helpmate and watchdog, trying to ensure that public policy protected and improved the lives of children and families. Maybe that was to remain my destiny as I crept through middle age, knowing that if I were lucky I'd have forty more years of a long life in which to cultivate other kinds of meaningful human connections. Having children wasn't the only way to give back to the world or to form unions with other warm-blooded mammals. I had become so focused on the notion of children that I had forgotten that other rewarding options existed. In fact, my slate was now squeaky clean. I had a whole new world in front of me.

Over the past year, I had allowed my old way of operating to completely slip away like a dead body sliding over the edge of a ship into dark deep waters. I became, in a sense, immobile. Not out of grief, because I did not feel grief over this new loss with Donor #2. I was too numb to feel grief. I was immobile because I was at a great crossroads. Biology was not dictating the course of my life as I had hoped it would. Ironically, for the first time in my life I had actually wanted my identity to be defined by my female biology. I wanted my daily routines to be dictated by an infant's needs rather than having to actively choose and construct a life. That was the root of my immobility. Infertility had defined and shaped our lives and identities for five years. In a sense, it had given us a purpose and a goal. I supposed I wasn't ready to let go of that goal just yet, still wasn't able to truly accept the fact that my body would not produce a child with my eggs or with someone else's.

❖

I suggested to Michael that we hunt through the photos on the donor website again. We could try another egg donor, and if that cycle didn't work we could try again. He looked at me with pity in his eyes. He had resigned himself to the fact that we had lost this round with Nature. Unless there was some lucky spell cast from the moon—perhaps a magic beam of light that would illuminate my ovaries at exactly the right second—we would remain a childless couple. I saw us growing old together, one of us dying in the other's arms, an eventual return to the earth. There were ghosts walking about who understood our hollow loss. Perhaps they were trying to tell us that our lives had to continue even if new life could not. I agreed, of course—but how? What did the future look like for a man and a woman exhausted from disappointment? That was the question we were now faced with, the task of reinventing the self, of reviving our relationship, of redefining our expectations. It had been done before and it would be done again, over and over, like the seasons, year in and year out. We were not unique, my fine husband and I. We were standing on the edge of something, but we didn't know what that edge was yet. Our quest for fertility had driven us further and further away from familiar surroundings. We now stood at a place where we had not stood before. Having nowhere else to place our feet, we had no choice but to jump and see where we might land.

LIFE CYCLES

When the leaves began to fall from the trees and the early cold winds of winter arrived, I began spending more time back at the farmhouse and I abruptly terminated my sessions with Susan.

"But we've done such good work these last few months," she told me gently. "We were just beginning to talk about adoption and how you might prepare yourself for that."

"I know," I said. "But that's a whole other giant mountain to climb. It's Mount Everest at the moment. I don't have the stamina or the oxygen supply, and I'm really, really tired of crying."

I hugged her goodbye and then, like the black bears that live in the state forest abutting our property, I slowly began to prepare for the winter hibernation period. I had to drag myself out of the house to teach or attend a yoga class or go out to dinner with friends. I was not capable of doing much else. I was barely functioning; my *joie de vivre* and that radiant glow I often emitted had dimmed. If I had been a caterpillar, I would have spun a soft oval cocoon around myself and hung suspended upside down from the ceiling all winter long, like a bat or a head of garlic in an Italian woman's kitchen. Babies hang upside down in their mother's wombs for weeks at a time during gestation. Perhaps my depression was actually a camouflaged rebirth, a shutting down of all my senses. Or maybe that was just wishful thinking.

By mid-January, I was in bed with a nasty chest cold that gripped my lungs like a vise for six weeks. No surprise, since I truly felt that life had been squeezed out of me. I welcomed the illness. It gave me a fabulous excuse to stay in bed for two weeks with my favorite black wool hat pulled down over my eyes to help me shut out the world. The winter landscape outside my bedroom window was stark and white and lifeless, a perfect reflection of my inner world.

I have long been a fan of director David Lean's masterpiece *Dr. Zhivago*, the famous love story set in Russia during the Bolshevik Revolution. You may recall the eerie winter scene where the desperate lovers take refuge in Yuri's summer home, ensconced in ice and snow and with a full moon hovering in the winter sky. We watch as a pack of hungry wolves paces and howls outside the house. For me, that scene more than any other conveys a sense of the vulnerability and fragility of life and love that stretch beyond the characters in the film. Whether we can admit it or not, we are all victims of fate and circumstance and nature. Some things in life are simply beyond our control, despite all the mind games we invent to pretend otherwise. Lying in bed during those two gloriously depressing weeks was liberating in a sense. My physical illness now matched my psychological state. I had no choice but to lie flat on my back, completely surrendered to life. I was too weak to stand. I had no appetite. My voice was gone. All systems were down, like the engine and lighting system failing in a plane that is 30,000 feet in the air. There was only free fall.

Anyone who has ever been ill understands that aggressively willing yourself back to health is futile. When you are sick—or when things aren't going the way you want them to go—you develop an edge of impatience. Frustration sets in. I hadn't realized it until then, but I was furious at my physical body. I was enraged at my ovaries for halting egg production. I was livid at my heart for bouncing into hormone-induced arrhythmia. I was angry that I was growing older. I desperately wanted to push the Pause button on my life. I knew enough not to push Rewind, but the Pause button would be nice. I needed a little bit of time to be completely still. I was forty-five years old. Half of my life had evaporated. Couldn't I please just have five or six months where I wouldn't grow another day older? Couldn't I take time to find my balance without suffering any consequences?

The answer of course was no. Life wouldn't wait for anyone. Either you leaped onto the spinning wheel and went along for the ride, or you stood on the sidelines and watched life pass you by. Up until now, I had been one of those people who had jumped on board and loved the speed of it all and the feeling of the wind in my face. Now I was content to just lie quietly in bed, like a corpse.

I was on the outside of my life now, looking in, the way one watches a bee that has been trapped inside a tall glass. This opportunity provided me with an unusual vantage point. I began to question why we humans spent so many hours in traffic jams and unproductive meetings with people we didn't necessarily like. Why were we sitting motionless for hours at a time in front of television sets watching reenactments of murders and rapes and robberies? Did our job promotions and professional titles really mean we were something other than what we saw in the mirror when we first woke up in the morning with bed head and bad breath? Was I any less of a woman for not bearing a child than the woman sitting next to me on the subway with four children in tow? Was Michael any less of a man for not being a biological father? All these ideas defined us because we *allowed* them to define us. But the ultimate question was, how do we define ourselves?

This was what I tried to figure out during my two weeks in bed, and what I concluded was that I didn't really care about some of the things I thought I did. I admitted to myself that I really didn't like spending time with people whose egos took up so much space there was no room left over for others to express their opinions. And I really didn't want to commute by train to New York City anymore and deal with the crowds in Penn Station. I realized that I had no desire to be nice to the nurse at the clinic because she really was a heartless robot of the greedy United States healthcare system, more concerned with her insurance payments than she was about me. What I did care about was sifting through all the layers of confusion I was feeling so I could stand on solid ground again. I needed to figure out if I wanted to adopt a baby or not.

❖

On a blustery February day, I watched as workers in a cemetery lowered a plain pine box into the frozen earth of New Jersey. My college friend Beth had died suddenly of an aneurysm. No one knew it was there until it ruptured and blood began to leak into her brain, slowly shutting down all her involuntary body functions.

She had been laughing with relatives at a cousin's birthday party one moment and then she had been transported by ambulance to the hospital. She died in less than twenty-four hours. Just like that, she was dead. There were no goodbyes. Just that harsh knowledge that no one would ever see her alive again. I pitied her husband and seven-year-old son. How would they make it through life without her? How would Andy find the strength to get up in the morning and not cry into the scrambled eggs he cooked for his little boy, who was the spitting image of his dead wife? How did anyone get through these tough times without crawling out onto the winter ice to escape the pain by freezing to death?

We humans are manufactured to endure incredible heartaches. Remarkably, the heart does heal and then it is ripped open again and then it heals, and that process continues until we die.

❖

Michael's father's health declined rapidly during the months between Thanksgiving and St. Patrick's Day. As his heart weakened and his strong fortitude faded, he began preparing himself and all of us for his impending death. The week before he took his last breath, he phoned me to say goodbye and to ask that I take good care of Michael and my mother-in-law.

"I will, Victor, I will. I promise. I love you." Exhausted, he whispered goodbye and hung up.

A few evenings later, Michael overheard him speaking with one of this home health aides during another sleepless night.

"Is there anything I can get for you, Mr. Victor?" the kind woman asked in her thick Caribbean accent.

"Yes," he replied. "Please make sure that Michael and Miriam have children."

Chronic heart failure chips away at a person's health and spirit in small doses over a long period of time. Victor escaped death more than once during his last decade, and with each episode he seemed to bounce back—never to 100 percent but enough to continue his bio-medical research and to enjoy his life and family. The day he died, he ate oatmeal for breakfast, and Michael half-carried him into the bath-room. He was weak, to be sure, but his death did not seem imminent. Because it seemed like any other day, Victor's passing taught me that the end of life did not mean that the gargoyles and the sleeping dragons came to escort yet another person to the Underworld. Death could be peaceful. Endings didn't always have to be jagged and abrupt.

We buried Victor four days later and grief wound tighter around us, like a python patiently waiting for the last breath to leave its prey. Michael and I committed even more intensely to becoming each other's loyal lifeguards; we kept a watchful eye on one another to ensure that we both stayed near the surface of our angst and did not slip beneath it.

At some point, every person on earth must come to terms with the notion that we are in some ways imprisoned by our mortality and in some ways liberated by it. Michael and I were beginning to realize that this was our moment. For some reason, I was comforted by the idea that the assimilation of this knowledge into our psyches was probably comparable to the first time Adam and Eve walked into a lake. I pictured them standing naked by the water's edge in Eden at sunrise, the cool air against their skin. The morning mist was rising off the water and small frogs sat quietly on bright green lily pads. Like them, I had finally realized that there was no separation between life and death; there really was no beginning, middle, or end. Life was a circle that expanded and contracted; some years were full and some years were empty.

❖

Michael and I knew that if we were going to build our family through adoption we had to remain proactive and drive the process forward, but we were both emotionally exhausted. The perseverance that had enabled us to hold on for so long during fertility treatments had walked offstage about the same time Michael's father died. We both feared that in our current state our long-held desire to become parents might fade away from us like a ship slowly drifting out to sea, growing smaller and smaller on the horizon until it was no longer visible to the human eye.

Somehow we found the strength to make an appointment with an adoption agency near the farm in western Massachusetts. I was cautious and not very talkative during our interview with the director; I was tired of strangers thinking they were entitled to ask us intimate questions about our lives. Besides, adoption agencies were also part of the booming baby business, and as businesses they had bottom line needs, just like the fertility industry. At this particular moment in my life, I didn't trust them; they were guilty until proven innocent.

In the wake of my silence, Michael spent half an hour filling in the blanks about our efforts over the last five years to create a family. I think for the first time he vented his rage about the failed science and the sadness he felt about losing his father. I sat quietly beside him and listened, nodding my head occasionally to show my agreement. When he was finished, the director took a deep breath and folded her hands on her desk, just as the Silver Fox had done during our first meeting at the clinic. Looking Michael straight in the eye, she informed us that adoption was not an easy path.

"I've been doing this for twenty years, and my gut instinct tells me that you aren't ready," she told us. "You are still too raw from everything you've gone through—from losing your option to have a biological child to losing your father. Why don't you two take a couple of months off and really think about whether you want to do this or not? And while you're waiting, I'd recommend you have some sessions with a counselor to help you cope with your grief and anger."

Wow. The director of this adoption agency had actually *rejected* us. We were stunned as we shuffled away from her office with our tails between our legs. She had actually deemed us unworthy of parenting. We weren't "allowed" to start the adoption process. Someone up in the heavens was playing really nasty tricks on us. Why was it so hard for us to become parents? What lessons were we being taught, and why?

"Sorry, babe," Michael said with a shrug of his shoulders as his eyes filled with tears. "I really screwed up this time."

"Shhh," I said, hugging him in the hallway. "It's okay. We're both pretty tired from everything we've been through. It's okay."

"It's too much," he kept whispering in my ear, the weight of his body surrendering into my embrace. "Maybe this is yet another omen to let us know that we aren't supposed to have children."

"Don't think that way," I replied in a soothing voice. "It's just too soon."

Secretly, I must confess, I was relieved that we didn't have to jump on board so quickly. Maybe it wasn't such a bad idea to pull back and figure out what our next steps might be.

"If we still want to have a family, adoption is the only way," Michael said to me the next morning. "I don't want to take any more time. That's all we did during treatments. It was a fucking waste of life. I am so angry that we spent five years doing that."

Ah, the glorious wisdom of hindsight.

I certainly shared Michael's sentiments. We were forty-five years old, and the clock was still ticking like the annoying drip of a leaking faucet. Each day we both grew more angry and frustrated; we felt constrained and strait-jacketed by all the events that were beyond our control. When we closed our eyes, we imagined how wonderful life would be in the future, when the passing of time would have filled all the gaping holes in our hearts. But we both knew this was an illusion.

In 1998, the revered Vietnamese Buddhist priest, Thich Nhat Hanh, said that the future was an imagined dimension of time, that the here and now was all that really exists:

> Let us not regret the past. Let us not worry about the future. Go back to the present moment and live deeply in the present moment. Because the present moment is the only moment where you can touch life. Life is available only in the present moment.

He was right, of course. We would invest so much time and energy longing for what we *thought* our lives should be like that we would lose track of what it *was* in the present moment. Staying anchored in our current depressing life was a tall order, but we had no choice. We were now confident that there was no such thing as greener pastures on the other side of the mountain.

❖

Trapped in the lonely eye of our post-fertility existence, Michael and I would wonder what happened to those incredibly carefree days of our thirties. There had always been so many friends to call at a moment's notice, trips to take, adventures to plan. Like millions of other couples in their thirties and forties, we desperately missed the company of old friends who had scattered across the country as a result of the double-edged employment diaspora that had afflicted our generation. Like those who came before us, our culture taught us that our professional achievements were what constituted a successful life. But our generation in particular had been assigned the job of mapping out how two-career families would cope with the logistical complexities of competitive job markets that economically rewarded those who were most mobile and versatile. Often we'd been asked to sever love relationships and give up the joys of living in a rooted community for promotions and bonuses. But the truth was, our disconnection from our lovers, friends, and families as a result of pursuing our careers had often caused us intense suffering. What was the benefit of a high-paying job if your quality of life was compromised and your best friends lived on the opposite coast?

One day a friend I hadn't spoken to in several years called me out of the blue, and I was glad I wasn't there to pick up the phone. The idea of having a "catch-up" conversation was the last thing in the world I wanted to do, so I sent her a card instead. I explained that I was sorry for having been out of communication for so long, but failed fertility treatments had stolen my tongue. Michael and I were both depressed, I told her. We were trying to pull ourselves up out of the thick mud that held us down. Maybe we could plan a reunion in a few months. I'd let her know.

In her efficient, pragmatic style, Jennifer immediately responded to my note with another phone call, which I also missed.

"I'm so sorry you and Michael are having such a hard time," she said in her message. "But couldn't we at least schedule a brief phone conversation so we can hear each other's voices and say hello? I really miss you and I want to know how I can help support you right now."

Tears welled up in my eyes when I heard her offerings of help. We hadn't spoken in so long, and the first words out of her mouth were, *What can I do for you?* She was such a good friend, in the truest sense of the word. Jennifer was the perfect example of the busy professional woman who had had the good sense to birth her two children at the ages the Silver Fox and the British Dr. Bewley had advised; she was finished with childbirth by the time she was thirty-three. She loved being a mother but had also been incredibly supportive and understanding of my hesitation to start a family of my own.

"You'll know when you're ready, if you are ever ready," she had said to me one day while she cradled her youngest son in her arms. "Motherhood is not for everyone, and you are the only one who can decide if that is true for you or not."

When we finally spoke by phone the following week, she let me know immediately that she understood what we were going through.

"I went through it myself in my early thirties," she told me as my mouth dropped open.

"I had no idea you went through that," I exclaimed.

"No one did," she said. "It was horrible and we were both miserable. I didn't tell anyone. Not a soul."

She had given birth to her first son when she was twenty-eight, and it had never occurred to me that so voluptuous and sexy and young a woman as she would have had trouble conceiving and birthing a second child. She and her husband tried multiple IUIs and one IVF cycle and then gave up. Their second son was conceived naturally two years later.

"Believe me, I know how hard it is to reel yourself back into the world," she told me. "I was *devastated*. I hated every minute of the treatments. The whole process was inhumane and humiliating."

I was discovering that many couples whose treatments had failed never wanted to talk about it—and who could blame them? There was a cultural taboo, reinforced by the clinics themselves, that said we shouldn't talk about our infertility or our miscarriages or the inability of science to solve our reproductive health challenges. It was this absence of truth telling that made the success stories sensationalized in the media so dangerously misleading.

When I told Jennifer we were thinking about adopting a baby, she—like everyone else we had begun to confide in—lit up like a bright light bulb.

"Oh, that's wonderful," she gushed. "I'm so happy for you. You and Michael will make wonderful parents."

We were not expecting such effervescent endorsements about our pending plans to adopt, but even strangers felt they had to add their two cents' worth of encouragement when they heard us talking about it.

"I know it's none of my business," an older woman in a coffee shop told us one morning. "But I have to tell you that adopting a baby is a blessing for everyone involved. If I could have children again I would, tomorrow, but I'm sixty years old now and it's out of the question.

My children are grown and I have six grandchildren, but still, if I could do it again I would. "

I wondered if she was aware of the fifty-six-year-old woman in Mansfield, Ohio, who had birthed her daughter's triplet babies. Maybe she would want to try that, too.

"Please don't mention that to her," Michael cautioned me with a raised eyebrow as he warmed his hands on his coffee mug. He hated talking about fertility, especially to strangers. He hated remembering the whole ordeal and how much time we had wasted. Now that his father was gone, he bore a double sense of loss that I could not even begin to fathom.

◆

The cynicism we harbored toward the fertility industry unfortunately spilled over into the world of adoption. We couldn't help it. Neither Michael nor I actually believed a real live baby would ever end up in our arms; the whole concept was now as abstract to us as a Disney cartoon. We had begun to really question whether we could emotionally afford to walk down that road again with no guaranteed outcome. Though the adoption agencies we interviewed reassured us about their placement track records, we had heard plenty of horror stories that were far from encouraging.

One friend had told us about a couple she knew who received a phone call at three in the morning from an agency wondering if they would be willing to adopt a retarded child with muscular dystrophy. There were birthparents who changed their minds hours before or after labor began. My gynecologist told me about two of her friends who actually *returned* their babies to the adoption agencies.

"I didn't know you could do that," I said.

"One was autistic and the other had been sexually abused and had serious emotional problems."

Gee, thanks for sharing.

One positive thing I was learning on this long journey toward parenthood was how to be a much more discriminating and discerning consumer. At this point in my life, I simply didn't believe what I was told or what I read. I was skeptical about adoption websites that boasted a three-month waiting period. Even in an agency with the best of intentions, a six-month wait could turn into a much longer journey. Adopting a baby was a gamble and a risk, just as fertility treatments had been. Babies died *in utero*. A pregnant woman could run away and never be heard from again. A dear friend could die from an aneurysm in her brain. There was still so much left to chance. Adoption was our new Casino Fertile but with different trimmings. It was a new deck of cards but still the same smell of a high-risk gamble was in the air, still the raw open wounds that come with being sucker punched so many times you couldn't stand up anymore.

❖

One morning I woke up with an idea that I believed was equivalent to Thomas Edison's invention of the light bulb. Why hadn't I embraced the idea of surrogacy earlier? Why couldn't we find a woman who was willing to have her eggs fertilized by Michael's sperm and then carry our half-biological child to term? Why had we wasted a year and a half and thousands of dollars on donor eggs, and now bogged ourselves down with adoption decisions, when we could have hired a surrogate?

I researched online and found an agency with an East Coast office. The staff person and I played phone tag for several weeks, and then she eventually e-mailed me some information. It was a price list, of course. There was nothing about success or failure rates and no information about how one coped emotionally with yet another bizarre high-tech reproductive process. The only tangible item I could hold onto was the big dollar signs—up to $75,000—for one try.

When I told Michael about my grand idea, he looked at me like I was mad. "There is no way in hell I'm going to do that. Enough is enough, Miriam. You have to let go of this."

"But there might be a woman out there somewhere who could provide us with eggs and an incubator. If we did it that way the child would be half you. *Half you.*"

"No," he said, getting visibly upset. "I am not going to rent some woman's body and buy her eggs. It's too much. I'm done."

I dropped it like a hot potato, and a couple of days later I realized he was right. We could go through the hell of that process and end up without a child, too. Adoption was the only way to go. But when I clicked onto my first adoption website I found myself right back in the place we had started with the egg donors: staring into the faces of strangers. The only difference now was that these strangers were cute little infants, toddlers, and adolescent children from all over the world.

I knew that many adoptive parents rejoiced in building a global family, adopting children from multiple ethnicities and celebrating their differences and similarities. Before fertility, from the outside looking in, I applauded their efforts and thought that maybe I would do that, too. But now that it was my turn, I froze. Here was yet another example of my privileged economic background allowing me to choose what kind of child I wanted to parent, as though I were deciding between a cashmere or mohair sweater. That nagging sensation of conspicuous consumption flared up in me again.

It was the same feeling that had weighed heavily on my heart when we were selecting an egg donor. Did we want a donor with a college education or a high school degree? Did we want a donor who was tall or short, buxom or flat-chested, skinny or plump? And when it came to choosing a baby, did we want a child with round or slanted eyes, white skin or brown, blonde hair or black? Here at the very beginning stages of investigating whether adoption was right for us, we once again felt uncomfortable about being in a position to choose our offspring's genetic traits. We were once again the all-powerful consumers with cash in hand, and for the right price we could bring an infant home with us.

◆

A week before Michael's father died, we had sat in a high school auditorium listening to a minister's wife from America's heartland talk about her journey toward becoming an adoptive parent. Late one night, a woman and four sleepy children had knocked on her front door.

"There is no room for us at the shelter," the distressed mother explained. "Please, can you take care of my children tonight?"

"Yes, of course," the minister's wife replied and ushered everyone inside, making up the couches and putting fresh sheets on the guest room beds. The children slept at her house that night, and the night after, and the night after that, until she realized that the mother was never coming back—that she couldn't come back—for any number of reasons. Maybe she was too poor to feed and clothe her children. Or perhaps she was involved in an abusive relationship and was afraid her children would be hurt.

"We knew the mother was obviously suffering enormous pain at not being able to care for her children," she explained. "We had to decide if we were going to call the Department of Social Services and deliver those children into a life of foster care or whether we would adopt them. We prayed on it and decided to raise them all as our own."

Only three minutes into telling her story, the dam inside of me broke loose and a river of tears began streaming down my face. My heart had cracked open again. This was the first time since we began this arduous baby-making odyssey that we were communing with people who actually talked about the sacredness of the path toward parenthood. Never once during all those years in treatment had anyone ever talked to us about or even mentioned the spiritual dimensions or ramifications of parenting new life.

"This is a very different group of people than we're used to dealing with," Michael whispered as he leaned over and handed me a tissue. "There is goodness and decency in this auditorium." I just looked at him, nodded my head in agreement, and tried as best I could to stifle the sobs convulsing through my body.

As the day wore on, we learned that this particular annual conference was always dedicated to the "triad of adoption": the child, the birthparents, and the adoptive parents. Experts discussed how interwoven this triad is in the emotional development of the child and how beneficial it is for children to know from an early age that they were adopted.

"You don't want your son or daughter to find out they are adopted when they are 11 or 12," one psychologist told us. "Or to find out from someone other than you. It's always best to be open, honest, and truthful in a child-appropriate way from an early age. Hiding anything from them, or avoiding any of your own grief about it, will only hurt the child."

We learned that it is not uncommon for adopted teenagers to perceive themselves as having two sets of parents, and that this can sometimes lead to confusion about their sense of identity and belonging. To counter their discomfort, adopted children may be more likely to disconnect from their adopted families and some may openly state that they wish another family could adopt them.

"I'm sure there are some differences between adopted versus non-adopted children in terms of emotional development," Michael responded when I shared the research with him, "but every teenager I've ever known wants to escape from their family—myself included." I loved this devil's advocate side of Michael's personality. Whenever someone tried to impress him with the statistics cited in some new study, he always asked who funded the research and tried to figure out an alternative methodology that might render different results.

"Please don't get bogged down in all the doomsday statistics about adopted kids running off and joining the Hare Krishnas," he advised me. "The most important thing we can do is love the child and let them know that they belong with us and that as long as we live we will support them and care for them."

In the afternoon, a social worker named Ellen led a workshop for couples recovering from failed fertility treatments. Of the *three-dozen* couples in the room, two stood up and shared their stories. One couple became pregnant after three years of treatments, only to lose that child in its sixth month. There was a deafening moment of silence underscored by a collective recognition of what such a loss must feel like. Michael and I had experienced one miscarriage—at seven weeks. The embryo was barely bigger than my pinky fingernail. This couple had actually had the opportunity to revel in the euphoria of their pregnancy. They had felt the baby kick in the womb and watched its heart beat on the monitor. Then one day it abruptly vanished, like Hiroshima after the bomb. There one day and gone the next. Talk about fucking with your reality.

The second couple had tried for *twelve years* to conceive. They were so driven to conceive a biological child that they took a second mortgage out on their house. This couple had surely crossed over into the Fertility Junkie Zone. They couldn't help themselves; their obsession had completely taken over their lives. I guess the wisdom of middle age or near-bankruptcy finally convinced them to step off the Fertility Merry-Go-Round and try adoption. Now in their mid-forties, they are the proud parents of three young African-American children. They spoke about the interracial dynamics of their family with a joy and a light in their eyes that I could not identify with. How could their eyes sparkle after all that? How could they possibly go through the laborious process of adoption not once but three times, and then, on top of that, cope with the incessant issues of racism they must encounter in their lives every day?

Halfway through the workshop, Ellen introduced us to Bob. He was a balding middle-aged man with a potbelly who just happened to be her adopted daughter's birthfather. They stood smiling side by side at the front of the room and told us that it was not uncommon for birthparents and adoptive parents to become friends. One of the couples that spoke told us they had spent their daughter's first Christmas with twenty members of her extended birth family in California. It was remarkable, really. One set of parents birthed a child they were unable to care for, and another set of parents that couldn't conceive stepped up to the plate to raise it. Then somehow they all form this convoluted community called a family. It made no sense and yet it made complete sense. Why not have both sets of parents involved in raising a child? Who was to say that one set of parents is better than two, or vice versa? Who made the rules when it came to family, anyway?

And what does it really mean to be a parent?

Could I only be a "real" parent if I birthed my own child, or was being a parent a role you acquired regardless of your biological connection to a child? Weren't the teachers all across America surrogate parents each day they taught a classroom full of children? Weren't school bus drivers surrogates, and the coaches who helped kids hit baseballs in Little League and score in a soccer game? Sitting there in that workshop, I began to realize that if we did pursue adoption, our assumptions about others and ourselves would once again begin to blur and likely disintegrate into nothingness. We would probably have to rebuild our identities and our ideas about the world from scratch, just as we had done when we moved deeper into the world of assisted reproductive technology.

A high school writing teacher of mine once tried to convey to me the Zen notion that the world is not as it appears. She did this by telling me the story of the Chinese master who showed his students a fish laid out on a platter.

"Write about this fish," the teacher instructed and the students did.

They described it as being ten inches long and three inches wide, with green and yellow flesh and beady black eyes. The teacher smiled when he read their assignments.

"What you have told me is how the fish looks on the outside," he told his students. "Now tell me about the fish."

The students were confused.

"Come children," the teacher said, "surely you can tell me where this fish was born and what rivers it has swum in. Where does it spawn? And what about the fisherman who caught it? Tell me this, students, and you will begin to understand that what we think we see and know is really just a figment of our own imagination."

JUMPING THROUGH HOOPS

One day in the late summer we met with a domestic adoption agency that didn't tell us to come back another time. Instead, they handed us a thick stack of forms to fill out and told us that, as soon as we cleared FBI criminal background checks and paid a fee of $500, the official process could begin.

They sure made it sound easy.

"Honey, I'll be right back with a baby," I thought to myself, wishing that it could be as simple as opening a package of Betty Crocker cake mix. Just pour the contents into a bowl, add one egg and some water—and voilà!

The truth was, those papers sat on our desks for weeks collecting dust and growing into a new kind of albatross around our necks. During the old days of trying to find an egg donor, we had at least been the ones in charge. We hunted through hundreds of photographs and profiles to find the "right" one. We were in control—or so we deluded ourselves—of our destiny and our child's future. But with adoption, the tables were completely turned; the birth parents had the right to choose us, we didn't choose them. I guess if I were in their shoes I'd want the same advantage. Couples who want to adopt are wallflowers waiting on the sidelines until birthparents invite them to dance. The adoptive parents' job is to wait patiently and hope the birthparents notice them.

Somehow Michael and I found the inner strength to pick up a pen and begin filling out the paperwork. Once we sent it in to the agency, they promptly assigned a social worker to our case. I had been fantasizing that ours would resemble Glenda, the Good Witch of the North. In my debilitated state, I desperately wanted to be mothered and cared for, but I was wishing on a star. Our social worker, Linda (not her real name), was a young woman recently out of graduate school, who was smart and thorough but not about to coddle me. During our first meeting with her, we listened as she described the nuances of the process we were getting ourselves into.

"It could take as little as four months or as long as a year or more, but in the end," she assured us, "you will definitely have a child."

"But you can't guarantee that to us, can you?" Michael asked skeptically. "I mean, we could wait another three years and spend thousands more dollars and still end up with no baby, just like we did with fertility treatments."

"Why does everyone think the adoption process will fall through? Our *job* is to place a child with you."

"Part of us thinks the adoption process will fail because we've heard stories about birthparents changing their minds at the last minute," I told her.

"That does happen," she said, "but not that often. Rest assured, you will become parents at the end of this process."

"We'll believe it when we see it," Michael muttered under his breath.

Linda explained that the Adoptive Parent Photo Album we needed to create was *the* most important communication tool linking us to the hundreds of birthparents out there in America who were coping with the challenge of choosing loving parents to raise their children. We realized then and there that now it was our turn to start thinking about ourselves as products, like a new hairspray or a computer. How could we convince a twenty-year-old birthmother that she should choose us? We had no idea.

While some couples seemed to enjoy making their album, I found it taxing. Intellectually, I understood that we needed to share our life story with the agency and prospective birthparents but I had a hard time wrapping my head around it emotionally. I was impatient and frustrated that we were still engaged in the process of "acquiring" a child.

"After everything we've already gone through, we now have to describe our worth as people and potential parents?" I ranted to Michael. "I am furious that we are allowing strangers to judge us and choose our destiny. I just can't stand it anymore."

"I know," Michael said, trying to soothe me and hold my hand. "But once again we don't have a choice. If we want to adopt a baby, we have to make this album. It's that simple."

"Right," I replied. "It's just like when we were doing treatments. What if we do everything the agency asks us to do and we still don't end up with a baby?"

"I don't know what we'll do," Michael said, shaking his head. "In some ways, I think this is our penance for waiting so long." Even though part of me agreed with him, I couldn't believe he had actually spoken those words. He sounded like a religious extremist who believed a diagnosis of infertility or HIV/AIDS was God's punishment for sinful thoughts or misconduct.

A few days later, when my anger finally subsided, we spread out hundreds of photographs of our life together on the dining room table. There was that great photo of us—taken *before fertility treatments*—at a friend's wedding in Chicago. We looked so incredibly happy; we were both literally glowing. It hurt to look at it now because we both knew that that radiance had dimmed a bit, and we were a little frightened that it may never return. We cried when we discovered an old photo of Michael's father, and another one of our dog, Luke, who had died only a year after we moved out to the farm. There were pictures of our niece and nephews when they were babies, and photos of them today in junior high school and college. We cringed at the passing of time on paper, and censored our urge to condemn the choices we had made individually and together. After moving in slow motion for two weeks, we finally pieced together a first draft of the photo album and showed it to Linda, who promptly rejected it.

"It doesn't seem to capture who you both really are," she said casually. "You are very earthy people, but it doesn't come across in the photos you have selected or the captions you have written. Why don't you go home and try again?"

Go home and try again? I was sick and tired of jumping through this endless corridor of hoops. In fact, I was so sick and tired of this whole mess of a life we had woven that I was tempted to punch holes in her office walls. Since the very day six years ago when we decided we wanted to become parents our efforts to make that happen never, ever seemed good enough.

"I'm sure the next draft will be more realistic," she said as she escorted me to the door.

I stood in the hallway outside her office and slowly slid down the wall into a squatting position. I bowed my head and took some deep breaths to shift my anger level down to neutral. I knew she was just doing her job. But she was young. What did she know about *life after fertility treatments*? Nothing really. She had no idea that Michael and

I still struggled with our desire to rediscover a post-fertility sexual-sensual connection free of sadness and guilt. And she really didn't know what it was like to wake up in the morning knowing that you could not change the current outcome and circumstances of your life. Her chances were not used up yet.

For days on end I couldn't shake the sense of livid rage that boiled inside me. A part of me still couldn't believe that we had once again placed ourselves in a passive role where we were relying on fate to chart the course of the family we wanted to build. Once again, we had selected a path whose outcome demanded that we completely surrender to the agency and trust their judgment, just as we had surrendered to the fertility industry. The notion of surrender nauseated me. I had given all my power away, and now I was doing it again.

A week later, the agency mailed us yet another stack of literature and forms to fill out. Like the previous ones, they also sat unopened for several days before we mustered up the nerve to review them. One of the new forms was a rather in-depth questionnaire they used to determine our comfort level with specific situations concerning the birthparents and their family history. The morning I settled into the couch with the paperwork and a cup of tea, I was optimistic. At my friend Meryl's suggestion, I had decided that I was going to stop making mountains out of molehills, do what was asked of me, and keep my eyes on the ultimate prize. But this strategy backfired immediately. The *very first question* asked how comfortable we were about adopting a baby that was born as the result of rape. What a wake-up call. Nothing was ever as it appeared. How could I have been so foolish as to think that we would adopt a baby from two teenagers who were playing doctor in a cornfield in Nebraska one afternoon and forgot to use a condom? How silly of me not to have thought about the millions of women and girls who become pregnant each year as a result of rape or incest. Whack.

The other questions inquired about our comfort level adopting a baby from a birthmother who drank alcohol or took drugs during her pregnancy, or who had a history of mental illness. How did we feel about adopting a baby if the father's identity was unknown? What about learning disabilities, criminal history, and diabetes? All the questions were difficult, but I kept going back to the rape question. How did I feel about adopting a baby that was conceived through violence? When the child was old enough to ask questions about his or her mother, was I supposed to be honest and admit the father was a rapist?

"Let's think about this for a second," Michael advised. "First of all, we don't have to tell the child that their mother was raped."

"If we want to be truthful and open with them, we do. Are you going to lie about it?"

"No. We don't need to lie, but we don't have to explain everything. If they are interested in discovering their birthparents when they are older that's their prerogative."

"And they'll ask why we never told them."

"And we'll respond that it was part of their personal journey to discover it on their own."

"It's horrible."

"Yes, all rape is horrible, but sometimes babies are born from date rape, which is still rape and violation, but not always as violent."

"So now we have to determine for ourselves what degrees of rape we deem acceptable and what ones we don't?"

"It sounds like that is what we have to do, yes."

During my next meeting with Linda, I asked her why the adoption agency had posed the rape question first. "I assume it's because you place a lot of babies who are conceived out of rape?"

"No, not at all," she replied. "Very few of our birthmothers have been raped."

"Then why would it be the very first question you pose on the questionnaire? It's a very jarring and upsetting way to begin the adoption process."

"Gee, I don't know. No one has ever raised the issue with us before."

I couldn't believe that I was the first person who became just a little upset by this question. Didn't other people speculate about how many of the seven billion humans who inhabit the planet were conceived through rape? Was I the only one who pondered how many babies were born in refugee camps or in war zones or in the stone houses that line the streets of Kabul?

Michael and I both wondered how many were born to parents who really didn't like each other and how many to parents who were madly in love. We had grown fascinated with the intriguing stories we had heard about how some babies were conceived. Our favorite was the two female professors at a small Midwestern college who engaged in an affair, only to be discovered by one of their husbands. Far from being upset, he invited himself into the bed. As fate would have it, this *ménage-à-trois* produced a child that was later placed for adoption.

Despite the gossip that lay behind the circumstances of every conception we heard about, we found ourselves asking the bigger question:

what really matters to us? If Glenda, the Good Witch of the North, delivered a brand new baby on our pillow one night would we automatically deliberate about the conditions of that child's conception? The answer was no. We'd immediately attend to the child and fall madly in love with her. The reason it mattered so much now was because our gestation period had expanded from the normal nine months to *six years*. We had nothing to do but wonder, spin stories, and worry.

❖

One day I received an e-mail from my friend who lived overseas. After *sixteen* failed fertility treatments—subsidized by her government's health care system—she had finally given birth to twins, who shared none of her or her husband's genetics. Their friends had donated frozen embryos, and, amazingly, they burrowed into her womb where they grew fat and healthy. She referred to it as "very early adoption." In the photo she cradled one baby in each arm, breastfeeding one while her husband bottle-fed the other.

Several days after the birth, the donors had visited them in the hospital.

"It was lovely," my friend reported. "We were nervous at first but they were so happy for us and so eager to see the twins."

I was dumbfounded when the technology actually worked.

❖

Linda called to remind us that it was time to schedule a meeting to discuss our preferences about our future child's racial and ethnic heritage. We squirmed with awkward misdirected resentment, knowing that if we had birthed our own child we would never have to engage in these disturbing conversations.

"Your comfort levels are the most important consideration during this discussion," she cautioned us. "If you aren't honest with yourself and each other, down the road there will be problems for the child. And no one wants that."

She was right, of course. The answers to these questions demanded grueling truth telling and exhaustive soul searching—individually and as a couple. This was not the time to imagine ourselves as *Superhuman Future Adoptive Parents* capable of handling any situation that was thrown at us. The fantasy might be that we would welcome any child in need—black, brown, or yellow—disabled, mentally ill, or diagnosed with disease. But we had been dragged over some rough terrain these last few years. The more realistic we were about what we felt we were capable of handling—emotionally and physically—the better off our child would be.

Linda established some ground rules before we began.

"If either one of you is uncomfortable with *any* of the hypothetical scenarios we discuss concerning the birthparents or their family histories, we cross it off the list—no questions asked. Does that sound fair and reasonable to you both?" she asked.

"Yes," we answered in unison. We had each browsed independently through the questions earlier in the week, and we knew we disagreed about some things. For example, Michael thought he would be comfortable raising an African-American child. As a dark-skinned man of Mediterranean descent, he had firsthand experience with racist barbs and knew what it felt like to be viewed as "other." He was fairly confident in his abilities to help a child from another race feel proud of his heritage and stand up for himself in challenging situations. I, on the other hand, was hesitant. When it came to race, I was not "other" in America. My fair-skinned, fair-haired appearance had never inhibited my ability to flow with the mainstream. My mother's WASP ancestors sailed over from England in the 1600s and settled on Cape Cod. If I wanted to, I could probably use this documented family lineage as a passport to joining the Daughters of the American Revolution. The point was, I had never personally felt the lonely isolation of racial otherness, and, unlike Barack Obama's mother, I was not sure I wanted to take on the complexities of raising a biracial family in a still racist America.

My close friends fiercely disagreed with my self-assessment and tried to convince me that I would be the *perfect* person for the job. But their endorsements were only proof to me that they had no concept of my current physical and emotional deficits, or my weaknesses as a human being. They knew me as an activist for social justice and human rights. They thought I'd uphold my brown-or-black-skinned child's dignity with ferocious determination each day of her life, and I probably would. But the truth was I was still exhausted from this baby-making marathon. I was weary—and leery—of fighting any more uphill battles. Right now I wanted the least complicated slice of the family pie that I could possibly have. Given all that, Michael and I checked the box next to "Caucasian" and decided that we were open to considering biracial situations on a case-by-case basis.

◆

A severe ice storm pummeled New England that winter and we lost power at the farmhouse for eight long, cold days and nights. It was forty degrees in the upstairs bedrooms and fifty-eight downstairs. We fried eggs on top of the wood stove that we kept blazing to prevent the pipes from freezing. As we automatically reached for light switches and thermostats that no longer functioned, we were reminded of just how much of our daily, industrialized lives we took for granted. Losing electricity made us realize how much our reliance on technology removed us from our primal, animal nature. Treatments had been sterile, formal, and dry; copulation was moist, warm, and wet. Why had I had placed so much faith in Petri dishes and drugs to make a baby?

One night after the power was restored I was channel surfing and came across a television program about a couple who had adopted a little girl with special needs. She had only one arm and her knees were bent in such a way that she resembled a crouching spider scampering across the surface of the earth. With help from her parents and teachers, this precocious little girl had discovered a vivid sense of herself by competing in and winning swimming tournaments. Of course, I wept through the whole program, partly out of deep admiration for the girl and her parents, but also because I knew I didn't have the constitution or the passionate desire one needed to parent a child with a disability.

I wanted to think that I was one of those special people who perform like saints in the face of adversity, who would adopt a dozen babies who were the products of rape simply because those children needed love and someone in their corner more than the next child might. I cried because that little girl was smiling. She was *happy* to be winning the race, and her parents and her coaches *loved* her—loved her spirit, loved her dedication, loved her no-nonsense I-am-here-on-this-planet-to-live-my-life-regardless-of-how-many-arms-I-have-and-how-crooked-God-may-have-made-my-legs.

"See me, I am here," her big smile said.

And I supposed I was here, too, in my muted, squandered spirit. The fertility treatments had maimed me. I was not quite as bold as I had been before, and that extra ounce of we-can-get-it-done attitude that I used to have had faded considerably. Perhaps it was a symptom of age, too; it was most certainly a symptom of defeat. Would the child we adopted change my mind about all of this? Would I begin to feel hope and a sense of optimism again once we held him or her in our arms? I wondered.

What I did know was that in the process of adoption, a child finds its way to its parents. It is not the other way around. The adoptive parents' job is to release control and open up to fate. It had some of the same sacred feeling that the birth story of Jesus had, or those myths about gods born to mortals. Not that I thought our child would be a messiah or a god, but I did in fact believe that all children and all people were Divine. We were all such works of art, such miracles. The fact that so many of us had come into this world at this one particular moment in time was mind-boggling. Most days it was too painful to think about; if you did consider each life precious, then the suffering we all experienced and inflicted and observed around us would be unbearable.

SHELL-SHOCKED

One morning I woke up angry as all hell. We'd been working on the second draft of our photo album for two weeks, and it still wasn't conveying an accurate picture of who we were. We didn't know how to convince a birthmother through photographs and captions that we were kind, trustworthy, caring people who would love her child with all our hearts. I was beginning to think that maybe we should go back to living our life the way we had before we became so obsessed with having children. We could sail around the world or live in Europe for several years. Maybe I could go back to school and study the art of writing comedy; I could turn our whole saga into a farcical film.

I was also upset with myself for passing judgment on the birthmothers of America, stereotyping them in my mind as drug addicts and women who were down and out of luck. The truth was, most of the women our agency worked with already had children of their own and they simply couldn't afford to raise another one. Others found themselves alone or in abusive relationships and knew their children would be better off in someone else's family. These women and men were selfless and courageous for placing their children with strangers like Michael and me, and all I could do was think about how the current economic downturn might actually be a boon to the adoption industry. I felt sick in my heart for thinking that I might benefit from another family's misfortune.

About the same time the economy tanked, my sister and I started to dismantle our parents' home. Since my father's second mild stroke several months earlier, my half-blind mother had made the decision to move into a new independent living complex one town away.

Rachel and I took turns transporting small pieces of their life into their new one-bedroom apartment. I supposed it was a retirement community, but it seemed more like a modern upgrade of the nursing home where my grandfather lived when I was a little girl. I recalled daffodil-yellow-and-white wallpaper in a wide hallway filled with dozens of old people lined up side-by-side in their wheelchairs. Day after day they sat there taking their medicines, eating their Jell-o, and waiting for death to claim them. One old woman with long white hair reminded me of a classic scary witch from Grimms' fairytales. She wore thick black horn-rimmed glasses and had a plethora of hairs on her chin. Every time we visited my grandfather, we had to walk past her wheelchair, and each and every time she called out to me.

"Girlie, girlie," she'd shout, as we cruised past her in single file like ducklings. "Come here, girlie, come here." I was ten years old and dumbfounded by her request for my company. Was I supposed to stop and say hello to her, or follow my dad into my grandfather's room where he was hallucinating about being back in Russia and hiding from the czar's soldiers during a raid on a Jewish village? I always opted for my grandfather's dementia.

With my parents' move to independent living, it dawned on me that they had actually grown old, too. My mother was still spry and cheerful, but my father was somber and beginning to move more slowly. Remarkably, he had retained his long-term habit of fighting against life—which may be part of the reason he was still alive after three bouts of cancer and two strokes. Like many elderly people, he had started taking an inventory of his life, and his remorse over my brother, in particular, seemed to overwhelm him.

Danny hovered on the edge of homelessness and financial instability, in large part because of the job discrimination he faced as an ex-offender. But he also had difficulty saving money for his future, and in fact I wasn't so sure he envisioned a future. When he told me he thought the bank might foreclose on his house, I became so panicked and scared for him that I decided to attend my first Al-Anon meeting.

I walked into a grand stone Episcopal church and listened as three women shared stories about their families. For the first time in many years, I felt an odd sense of relief that I was not the only one who had a troubled sibling I could not fix. When it was my turn to speak, I told them that Danny was in economic crisis almost weekly and, now that my parents could no longer afford to send him money, my sister and I were concerned that he might turn to drugs again, or end up back in jail or in a homeless shelter. I was pained by his instability. I didn't know what to do.

"There is nothing you can do," the first women who spoke told me gently. "He is the one who has to choose, not you. You have no control over the situation."

There it was again, that phrase, that notion that I had no control. How many times was I going to dupe myself into thinking that I had any power over my life or someone else's? Yes, I could choose whether to order a tuna or egg salad sandwich at the deli, but beyond choices like that, how much control do we really have? Not much, as the tenets of Alcoholics Anonymous clearly stated.

It was in that church basement that a very old woman whose alcoholic father was long since buried in the earth turned to me with her deep blue eyes and helped me understand that AA's interpretation of "Higher Power" was not necessarily one of a God up in heaven.

"I used to think Higher Power meant up there," she said, pointing her arthritic index finger toward the ceiling. "The fact is, as I deal with my daughter's mental illness and my other daughter's retardation, I realize time and time again that Higher Power, at least for me, means the interventions of fate and the help I receive through other people. For me, the notion of Higher Power shows up through circumstance and serendipity."

Circumstance and serendipity—that's what the adoption process was all about, too.

❖

I couldn't help it. Most mornings I woke up raging at myself, the fertility industry, and my parents with such anger in my heart that I thought blood would spurt out of my ears. I would spit and strike out like a rattlesnake, and there was nothing anyone could do or say to make me feel better. My yoga practice took the edge off temporarily, but inevitably the anger crept back. Figuring out how to exorcise this recurring wrath eluded me, like a fast-flying bird I saw only for a second before it rustled its wings and flew away. Whatever it was played hide-and-go-seek, and then sneaked into my bed at night to wake me. The Season of Insomnia had returned to torture me again.

During waking hours, I was engaged in a constant, conscious exercise of weighing the good with the bad, of striking a balance. I was filled with hate and love, joy and dread, fear and adventure—all at the same time. Finding equilibrium in the midst of this series of frenzied emotions was not easy. I was antsy and jittery. I worried about my parents' health and about Michael. I worried about my mother-in-law's loneliness since her husband died and about Barack Obama being assassinated. I worried about Israel and Hamas, Iran and Pakistan, and the threat of a nuclear war. I worried about the economic crisis and jobs and that thing called national security that I knew didn't really exist. Anxiety spread over me like a silk shawl and nestled into the crevices of my brain. I so desperately wanted to feel that limitless optimism I used to feel but I kept slipping back again and again into the dismal abyss. If I could just wrap my head around that notion of acceptance that Thich Nhat Hanh talked about, I knew I'd feel better, but it seemed that I couldn't reach acceptance until I burned through this blinding rage.

My fury reminded me of the five stages of grief, outlined in the 1969 book *On Death and Dying*, by the Swiss psychiatrist Elizabeth Kübler-Ross: denial, anger, bargaining, depression, and acceptance. There is no doubt in my heart that Michael and I experienced each of these phases individually and as a couple during treatments, and even now, since we have turned away from them. Our initial pursuit of assisted reproductive technology clearly marked our deep psychological need to deny the painful verdict of our infertility. When the science first failed us, we raged at the world and ourselves, and then sank into a deeper kind of denial, one laced with a dash of bargaining to ward off the impending depression that loomed like a dark thunderhead.

This is the phase that earns the global fertility industry its multi-billion-dollar annual income. I call it the Let's-Just-Do-One-More-Cycle Phase. It lasts the longest and can bankrupt many couples in all sorts of ways unless they have the mental clarity and emotional where-withal to push the eject button. Having now stopped treatments completely, we were still slogging our way through the endless swamplands of "anger," "depression," and "acceptance." We both wondered how long it would take for us to reach the acceptance phase and how many other couples were going through the same hard times.

Our friends who adopted a child after five years of failed treatments—including the loss of twins, one at six months—told us that as soon as they held their daughter in their arms the grieving life they had known just vanished.

"I know that whatever we say to you right now won't make sense because it all feels so abstract," Joe told us one night. "But believe me, all the anguish, regrets, and losses will fade away. It's something you'll have to experience to believe, and right now, I'm sorry to say, all you can really do is persevere."

Michael looked remote and somewhat dazed as he listened to our friends describe their first few weeks of parenthood. He seemed so fragile. If Kübler-Ross were still alive, she could launch a whole new branch of research into the five stages of grief associated with surviving failed fertility treatments.

❖

After weeks of home visits, piles of paperwork, and three photo album drafts, Linda finally granted us official approval.

"What exactly does that mean?" Michael asked.

"It means that you are now 'waiting parents' and that we send your album out to birthparents who match your preferences and vice versa."

"How long do you think we'll have to wait until we are matched?" he asked, stealing a glance at me.

Since we had completed all the requirements for the agency, we both felt that a great weight had been lifted off our shoulders. We had talked the night before about how important it was to stay focused in the here and now and not drift away with thoughts about the future. Could we just live our life *normally* now, knowing that one day the phone might ring and we would instantly become parents? It took as much emotional and intellectual fortitude and awareness to stay balanced in the limbo of adoption as it did to stay intact during fertility treatments.

"Well, there's no way to predict how long it will take to be matched," Linda said. "Sometimes it takes three months, sometimes a year, and sometimes longer. But don't worry—you will be matched. We are going to talk about that in the adoptive parenting class that starts next month. It will run for six sessions every other week, and we'll answer all your questions. There are eight other couples like you who are waiting. It will be fun and supportive."

Well, fun and supportive sounded good to us. It would be nice to take a break from the tightrope of emotional tension we had both been feeling. Michael was lucky. He had busy days to distract him, but I didn't know anyone in Boston. I occupied my time by going on job interviews, but in the slumping economy no one seemed to be hiring. On some level, it didn't even matter—who would want to hire someone as emotionally wrecked as I was?

Several days earlier, we had interviewed a local pediatrician the agency had recommended to us. It felt more than a little strange to walk into her office without a baby in tow and ask her questions that seemed so irrelevant to our existence in the present moment. Why were we discussing diaper rash and colic when we didn't even have a baby? Inside it felt like we were living a make-believe life and that this interview was part of a fictional script.

The doctor greeted us with a big smile and a warm handshake. She said she worked with many families adopting children and would be happy to be our medical consultant during the matching process. I did everything in my power to hide my sadness, but she was an astute observer.

"Are you okay?" she asked.

"Yes," I replied. "This is hard."

"I know," she said empathetically. "I'm assuming you went through fertility treatments?"

"Five years' worth," Michael said with a deep sigh.

"You're not alone," she told us. "There are so many couples adopting children now because the treatments didn't work for them."

"We even tried donor eggs," Michael said.

"And that obviously didn't work."

"No. In fact, the doctors deemed our two donors infertile."

"Your donors were infertile?"

"Yes, they were both infertile," I said softly. "There are no laws requiring the agencies to screen them ahead of time."

"No wonder you're ready to burst into tears. Would you like a tissue?"

◆

"You're a pressure cooker," Michael said to me one evening. "You need a shot of vodka to relax."

"I don't want to drink alcohol to relax," I told him. "I want to figure out why this poltergeist has colonized my body."

"Well, don't you think it has something to do with the fact that your dad had a second stroke and now you're packing up your parents' house?"

"Yes."

"And don't you think it has something to do with the fact that it's been six years and we still don't have a child?"

"Yes."

"And you don't have a job?"

"Yes."

"And my dad died."

"Yes. Yes. Yes. What's your point?"

"My point is that you have a lot on your emotional plate. You need to cut yourself some slack."

Cut myself some slack. Easier said than done when your own mind was holding you hostage.

But, as fate would have it, several days later a friend sent me an announcement for a conference about "Attachment, Trauma and the Body." It was geared toward social workers and psychologists but I was drawn to it hoping to find some clue as to how I might unlock the iron fist that settled in my belly every morning when the sun rose. That first day we watched captivating film footage of soldiers from four different wars who were afflicted with post-traumatic stress disorder (PTSD). There was a disturbing clip of a World War I veteran talking and laughing in his hospital room. He appeared perfectly healthy and happy until a nurse clapped her hands near his ears—an action that sent the poor man into such a fit of terror that he dove under his bed for cover. Years after the armistice had been signed, the former soldier was still unable to distinguish his foxhole experiences from his life in postwar America.

Dr. Bessel van der Kolk, the world-renowned psychiatrist presenting the lecture, explained the various kinds of therapies that had been used over the years to treat military and civilian patients living with severe trauma. One treatment was called Eye Movement Desensitization and Reprocessing (EMDR), a modality developed by Dr. Francine Shapiro that required patients to move their eyes back and forth while thinking about particularly difficult events in their lives. Scientists believed that the bilateral movement of the eyes during EMDR sessions liberated traumatic experiences from one region of the brain and allowed them to be reintegrated in a less intense state in a different area. Under normal stresses most people were able to process their negative memories through talk therapy or even through their dreams. But sometimes, for any variety of reasons, the event might replay over and over again, the way a CD player might become stuck and repeatedly play the same line of a song. Even after many years have passed, the level of intensity or panic that a particular trauma might have initially caused a person can remain the same.

Dr. van der Kolk showed us "before" and "after" videos of a woman who had been in a terrible car accident. On the first day of treatment she appeared to be literally frozen inside her body: her shoulders were hunched up around her ears and she barely seemed to be breathing. Like the World War I veteran, her existence was one of intense fear and terror; months after her accident she was still trapped inside her car. After three EMDR sessions, the woman looked like a different person. She was relaxed and happy and smiling. When asked about the accident, she waved her hand at the counselor as if to say, "Oh that little incident? Well, that happened a while ago and I've since moved on."

Could EMDR really be so effective that only three sessions could untangle a person's tightly wound nervous system? It sounded too good to be true, but I actually knew several people who raved about it. When my friend Bonnie was thrown from a horse several years ago, she was afraid to get back in the saddle again.

"You know how much I love horses," she told me. "I live and breathe horses but I couldn't for the life of me imagine riding again." A feisty mare had reared up on its hind legs and bucked her backside onto the hard earth of Colorado. She broke two ribs, cracked a lumbar vertebra, and suffered a dozen other injuries. A year after her physical body healed, she knew she was ready to tackle her psychic wounds.

"I did four EMDR sessions," she told me, "and now I'm riding again. I'm cautious and a bit fearful, but I'm riding again three times a week."

Another man I knew told me that EMDR had completely transformed his life. "I was able to sleep through the night for the first time in years," he explained with a big smile. "I had been plagued by insomnia for more than a decade."

Maybe it was too good to be true, but I figured I had nothing to lose by trying, so I made an appointment with Dr. van der Kolk.

❖

I had been acutely anxious, depressed, and teary every day for almost four months, and when I arrived at his office I was literally ready to jump out of my skin. I would have traded bodies with anyone willing to swap; I was so stuck in my trauma grooves that I really thought I would never be happy again. I dumped my entire plate full of problematic lifetime events into his lap during that first session. We talked about the huge disappointments of fertility treatments, my concern for Danny, and lingering hurts from childhood that had come back to life when I started spending so much time at my parents' house. He watched my body for clues about my past; when I stopped breathing or my face became flushed he'd ask me to pause and take a deep breath.

"Can you be still for a moment?" Dr. van der Kolk asked in a soothing voice. "Can you be still and observe the sensations you are feeling in your body right now?"

"I have a pit in my stomach, and my thighs feel very tense," I replied in a small voice. "My legs feel very heavy."

"Okay," he said. "Now I want you to watch my index finger. Track the movement of my finger with your eyes and take a deep breath."

I did.

"Keep watching my finger," he said gently. By the end of sixty seconds, I felt a radical shift in my physical body. There was a pressure behind my forehead and the tension in my legs and belly turned into waves of heat and energy that moved up and down my thighs. I smiled.

"Why are you smiling?" he asked.

"Because I am having the opposite feeling than I had before you waved your finger."

"Good," he said. "Good."

In that instant, I felt a joy I had not felt in a very long time. I was no longer plagued by those heavy physical feelings of doom and gloom and victimization. I was as close to just being in the moment as I had ever been in my life. There was no need to run, cry, rage, or grieve. I could just sit in that chair in that office with that doctor and breathe. We did four mini-EMDR sessions during my first meeting with him, and I truly did feel like I had a new lease on life. So much of the heavy anxiety I had been carrying melted away.

"Oh, my God," Michael said to me one morning several days later.

"What?" I asked.

"You're smiling."

"I am?"

"Yes, you're smiling again. Thank God for EMDR," he said as he gave me a hug and a kiss.

I continued EMDR sessions with a different therapist—ironically, with a woman who during our first meeting told me that she had gone through fertility treatments fourteen years earlier and successfully birthed a daughter. Now that my body was beginning to calm down, I could see that the discomfort I had endured for so many months had actually been a well-camouflaged gift. Mornings were now transformed into symbolic opportunities for rebirth and creativity, and I began to appreciate the wonderful people in my life. A dozen dawns in a row I observed the subtle sensations that arose when crossing over from a dream state to wakeful consciousness. At home at the farmhouse, I reveled in the luxury of lying next to Michael while he slept, studying the contented expression on his face. I watched the play of light on the clouds and the mountains as the darkness of night receded and the brightness of the day unfurled. I listened to the melodic sounds of the mourning doves as they perched high in the tree outside our bedroom window. I realized that I was indeed on the road to genuine happiness again.

❖

There were sixteen people in our adoptive parenting class, and every single one was a Fertility Refugee with varying degrees of scar tissue and trauma to show for it. We were the middle-class guinea pigs of our generation who had donated our bodies to science and ended up with the short end of the stick. Like Michael and me, our classmates exhibited a shell-shocked quality in their body postures and facial expressions. I recognized in them what was true for me: that sadness in the eyes and the slight downturn of the mouth.

A recent study by Allyson Bradow from Spalding University, *Primary and Secondary Infertility and Post-Traumatic Stress Disorder*, revealed that women who experience failed fertility treatments often found the situation so distressing that they developed PTSD. Close to 50 percent of 142 participants met the official criteria for the disorder—about six times higher than the percentage of people in the general population. Common symptoms included feeling distant or cut off from people, irritable, anxious, and hopeless. In an odd way, it was comforting to know that Michael and I were not the only ones who still felt off-balance after the treatments.

Until I met this particular group of men and women, I had not realized how alone I had felt and for how long. Early on in our epic journey I had researched RESOLVE and the American Fertility Association—the nation's two most popular support and advocacy groups for infertile couples. Perhaps I would have felt better had I attended a meeting or two, but I never felt quite comfortable reaching out to them because they receive funding from pharmaceutical companies and fertility clinics. I thought their perspective might not be that different from that of the social workers who worked at our clinic.

Over the years my friends had provided me with generous support and love, but they could not truly understand the devastating losses that infertility dredges up in one's soul. This group of Fertility Refugees did understand. While other generations shared legendary cultural moments like Woodstock and Burning Man, a growing number of my generation were bound through our experiences with reproductive technology. Everyone in that room had endured multiple cycles, some more than others. Collectively, we had spent millions of dollars and wasted decades of our lives trying to make babies in laboratories. And now we were huddled together in the adoption office, plodding along the dotted lines of yet another abstract map that we hoped would lead us to the children we could never birth ourselves.

During one class, the agency arranged for us to meet two sets of adoptive parents and their beautiful babies. Little three-month-old Isaac was sitting on his mother's lap next to Michael and managed to maintain eye contact for quite some time—long enough for Michael to realize something he hadn't known about himself before.

"I love that kid," he told me after class. "Did you see him? I'd bring him home with me in a heartbeat. When are we getting our baby?" I smiled. The man who was worried about his ability to love was smitten in less than thirty minutes.

Baby Night was probably the hardest class for all of us refugees to sit through; most of my classmates were slumped in their chairs with their arms and legs crossed, subconsciously protecting themselves. Though I'm sure the agency thought it would cheer us up to know that real live babies do actually get matched with real live couples, the presence of the babies seemed to push everyone's buttons. One woman sitting across from me was nearly in tears. After class, I asked her if I could give her a hug.

"Why would you do that?"

"Because I thought you needed one about an hour ago," I told her. "I saw that you were very sad."

I hugged her, and then she started to cry. "I can't stand this process," she told me as a big tear rolled down her left cheek. "I can't stand the waiting."

"You sound just like me," I said.

"We haven't even started making our photo album," she confessed in a frustrated voice. "On top of all of the heartache we went through with the fertility treatments, the adoption agency is now asking us to tap dance and hang upside down from a high wire. When does it end? When do we just go home with a baby in our arms and live a normal life like everyone else?"

Michael and her husband stood quietly nearby and watched while she did a little tap dance and then took a bow. The hint of a smile replaced her tears, and we all chatted in the parking lot for another half hour.

❖

A few weeks later, on the recommendation of one of the couples in our class, I found myself alone for the first time in the baby section of a department store.

"It's a good idea to stock up on basic items like diapers, wipes, and blankets," they had advised me. "You never know when the phone might ring."

That was true. We had no idea when and if the phone would ever ring, but here I was, the barren older woman standing in front of a baby carriage that resembled a piece of the Space Shuttle. Feeling awkward and somewhat terrified, I made my way through each aisle placing various baby sundries into my shopping cart. I stopped in the diaper aisle to watch a thirty-something mom interact with her infant.

"How old is your baby?" I asked, practicing for the future mom-to-mom interactions that so many of my friends with children had told me about.

"This is Ashley," the women replied. "She's six months old today."

"Hi, Ashley," I cooed, bending down and peering into a mass of polka-dotted blankets that framed the baby's face.

"When are you due?" she asked, spying the mound of baby supplies in my carriage.

"Well, I don't know," I told her with a little laugh. "My husband and I are adopting."

"Oh, congratulations," she replied with a big bright smile on her face. "My sister is looking into adoption. She went through fertility treatments but they didn't work."

"We tried that, too," I told her.

"Well, it's still a very young science," the woman said. "And very little research has been funded and conducted. I'm actually a fertility researcher."

"Really?"

"Yes, I study which treatments and procedures are more apt to increase ovulation and sperm count."

"Can I ask you a question?"

"Of course."

"Do the clinics gather research from their customer base? I mean, if they don't have grants to conduct controlled studies, I assume that they might try certain drug combinations with their patients, track their success and failure rates, and then compare results across patients."

"I obviously can't speak for the whole industry but I certainly have relied on internal data from my clinic for my research projects," she said. "The pharmaceutical companies work closely with clinics to determine which drugs work best to offset certain symptoms of infertility. Right now, the greatest success rates across the board are with women under thirty-five."

"Well, yes, I've heard that's true for IVF cycles," I said. "But what about donor eggs?"

"Our clinic has a cut-off age of forty-two for IVF and donor eggs. Once you are past that age success is very rare, even for donated eggs."

"But we started at our clinic when I was forty-two," I said, feeling even more naive than I did before. "Our clinic's cut-off age for IVF and donor eggs was fifty."

"Well, most clinics won't tell you that you don't stand a chance," she said.

Her words stung my face like sleet in a storm. I drove home feeling more gullible than ever for having succumbed to the seductions of the industry's excellent marketing schemes. I took some comfort in knowing that every man and woman in my adoptive parents class probably felt the way that I did, and that some of Michael's friends from high school did, too.

At his recent class reunion, without his even mentioning our story to them, six women friends he hadn't seen in twenty years confided in him about their failed treatments.

"We are the Gypped Generation," one friend from California said. "They told us that we didn't have to rush to have kids. They told us it was okay to wait, and in the end it's not. If I had known that the technology had such a high failure rate, I *never* would have waited. I would have happily had children earlier if I knew there was no other alternative. I feel like they lied to us."

RENEWAL

In April I drove out to the farmhouse by myself for several days of peace and quiet. Our illusory city escape was now a full-fledged construction site. There were a dozen sub-contractors banging away on all four floors, installing new windows and kitchens and bathrooms. I thought that surrounding myself with the early sights and sounds of spring might help me cast off the heavy cloak of victimhood I had grown so accustomed to wearing. Several close friends had expressed deep concern about my lingering sorry state and wondered what it would take for me to crawl back up into the sunlight.

"I don't know," I told my friend Bonnie when she flew in from Colorado for a brief weekend visit.

"What do you mean, you don't know?" she asked in that half-sarcastic, half-loving voice of hers. "You're Miriam Zoll. You always have a plan of action."

"Not anymore," I confessed as my throat choked off my words. "I don't know anything anymore."

"You, my dear, are feeling sorry for yourself. You have so much to be grateful for. Don't you know that?"

I looked at her the way a deer stares into the headlights of an approaching car at night: I had absolutely no idea what she was talking about. What aspect of my wretched post-fertility existence could possibly look like something I should be grateful for? The EMDR had helped me to a certain degree but it was no panacea. We were living part-time in the dark and depressing basement unit of an apartment building until the full renovation was complete. We still had no child. I was currently unemployed, and, on top of that, all the beliefs I had held to be true about the world and myself no longer applied. I had no solid ground to stand on.

"Well, for starters," Bonnie said, "you don't live in a war zone and you're not starving. You keep talking about being a Fertility Refugee but compare your privileged life to a real refugee, say a woman living in the Congo whose entire family has been murdered. She's now residing in a Red Cross tent city with 10,000 other people who are homeless and plagued by night terrors. That woman has problems you can't even begin to imagine."

"Okay, okay," I said, feeling threatened and defensive that she was trying to take my familiar woe-is-me mindset away from me. "But I have gone through hell, you know. You have no idea. It's only recently that I've even been able to get out of bed in the morning."

"I know you've been having a hard time," she said, "and please know that I am not in any way trying to deny you your experience. But after thirty years of friendship, what I do know about you is that you are not a victim. You are a brave and courageous woman, and in less than a year you are going to become a mother. It's time to start rising up out of the muck and start walking on land again. You need to find your feet and walk away from this episode. It's over, but you're still acting like it's not."

Bonnie and I had become fast friends when we met in the seventh grade. Her family was just as bizarre and troubled as mine, and all through our adolescence we relied on each other to stay sane. Our phone conversations were always direct and to the point, and the few precious face-to-face visits we'd had since she moved out West were always filled with sharp and insightful observations about each other's lives. Because she was my oldest friend in the world, Bonnie was allowed to employ tough-love tactics with me when necessary to kick my ass into gear. On this particular visit she skillfully held the mirror up to my face so I could see and hear the self-pitying woman I had become.

◆

During the drive out to the house, I listened to a story on National Public Radio about a former high school football player named Ed who was plagued by an extreme case of Obsessive-Compulsive Disorder (OCD). At the age of eleven, he had watched his mother die—an event so traumatic that he began inventing complicated rituals he subconsciously hoped would freeze or reverse time and bring her back to life. If he ate a plate of spaghetti without letting a strand of it land on his chin he might be able to freeze six hours of time, which he acknowledged by tapping his cheekbone six times with his index finger. But if a strand of spaghetti did touch his chin that meant he had to do something entirely different, like count to 16,000 by doubling numbers—2, 4, 8, 16, 32, all the way up to 16,000—which he did several times a day.

His affliction grew worse as he grew older, to the point where he eventually cloistered himself in his basement for two solid years. During that time, he never bathed or went outside for a walk. His worried family tried various kinds of unsuccessful interventions until they finally located an OCD psychiatric expert who agreed to meet with him in person. Over the next several years, Ed made small strides here and there, but his recovery was still painstakingly slow. Some months, every step forward meant three steps backward. One day, feeling completely powerless about his patient's lack of progress, his doctor suddenly broke down in tears.

"What's wrong, Doc?" Ed asked with alarm.

"I've tried everything I can think of to help you," he replied in a sad and exacerbated voice. "I desperately want you to live your life again. You are a wonderful, caring man. Your sensitivity astounds me. But nothing I do seems to be helping you. Drug therapy doesn't work. Behavior modification doesn't work. I just don't know what to do for you anymore."

Ed watched in detached silence as the doctor cried, observing him the way a tourist might study the behaviors of a monkey or a polar bear in a zoo. Then he had one of those "Aha" moments that ultimately transformed his life in the blink of an eye.

"I was so touched that the doctor was crying for *me*," Ed explained, "so moved by his compassionate desire for me to have my life back, that I decided right then and there that I was not going to let the OCD rule my life anymore. *I chose my life over my illness.*"

Tears were streaming down my face as I listened to Ed describe the agony of his former existence. He had been down and out and close to a spiritual if not physical death when the doctor opened the door and let the fresh air flood his lungs and the sunlight blind his eyes. The magic word in Ed's story was *choice*—that remarkable human gift that enables us to select what kind of book we read or dinner we eat or thoughts we think. It had taken years for Ed to harvest the strength and courage he needed to push his disorder into the background of his life, but with time and grace and companionship he had finally succeeded.

His story reminded me of a passage from a well-worn book I had bought years before when I first started practicing yoga. The revered Tibetan Buddhist teacher Chogyam Trungpa Rinpoche wrote *Shambhala: The Sacred Path of the Warrior* to help people reconnect to the principles of living the sacred and dignified path of the warrior. The word "warrior" in this context was taken from the Tibetan word *pawo*, meaning "one who was brave." Trungpa wrote about the transformation that occurs when a warrior freed himself from the World of the Setting Sun and embraced the Dawn of the Great Eastern Sun:

> The way of cowardice is to embed ourselves in a cocoon in which we perpetuate our habitual patterns. When we are constantly recreating our basic patterns of behavior and thought we never have to leap into fresh air or onto fresh ground. The Dawn of the Great Eastern Sun is based on actual experience. It is not a concept. You realize that you can uplift yourself, that you can appreciate your existence as a human being. Whether you are a gas station attendant or the president of your country doesn't really matter. When you experience the goodness of being alive, you can respect who and what you are.

It seemed to me that Ed and I were both warriors who had lost our way. We were once powerful people, but our disorders and depressions had eclipsed the light that had illuminated our path. Recognizing that we even had a choice to make was the first step in unlocking ourselves from the self-manufactured cages we inhabited.

A wise woman I had known for a brief time when I was in my early twenties had one day tried to explain to me that "you get what you speak about."

"So talk about love, not hate, and joy, not fear," she explained with a big smile. "Your words and your thoughts create your life. You have the power to control what you think about and what manifests in your life."

It sounded like mumbo-jumbo to me back then, but now I knew exactly what she was talking about. Her message was the same as Ed's: we all have the power to choose what thoughts we nurture and which ones we dismiss, and depending on our life circumstances some of us have to work longer and harder to achieve this state.

While listening to the radio in the car that day, I had an "Aha" moment, too. I realized that I was finally ready to at least try to *accept* my past without being branded or defined by it. It was time to integrate the truth about the choices I had made—all of them, the good and the bad, the sad and the happy—into one body and one mind and one life. Like a well-trained and disciplined warrior, I knew I possessed the emotional tools and the personal power to proactively reclaim my life. Enough tears had been shed. It was time to start looking forward again.

❖

Springtime at the farmhouse was always a dazzling spectacle of nature. When I arrived, the sun was lighting up the mountainside and the first traces of green and purple buds were glowing against a lavender-blue sky. A light dusting of snow still covered the grass and the fields, and I smiled when I heard the chatter of the songbirds that had recently returned from their winter nesting grounds. The peepers—those tiny frogs with vocal chords as big and powerful as Pavarotti's—had already started crooning their love songs to prospective mates. By late April and early May their collective croaking would be so deafening we would have to cover our ears with both hands as we passed them on our evening walk. I was most happy and relieved to see that a small patch of yellow and purple crocuses by the side of the front porch had already bloomed. Every spring I waited with great anticipation for these tiny flowers to thrust themselves up through the cold earth into the sunlight. They were like reliable lighthouses signaling to all who cared to notice that the seasons and cycles of life always moved forward, even when we thought we couldn't.

Later, I walked into the fields that Michael and I had cleared when we first moved into the house years before. Back then, hundreds of young pine trees had colonized the land that generations of New England farmers had toiled over so that cows might graze and crops might grow. We used to race into the fields on our blue tractor, rev the engine, lower the bucket to almost ground level, and drive full-speed into the trunk of a tree. Once we flattened it, we'd wrap it in a heavy chain, lift the bucket up toward the heavens and pop the roots out of the ground. We'd stack the trees into piles and burn them on rainy Saturday afternoons.

After checking to see if there were any small snakes or voles, I lay down on my back in the tall grass with my arms stretched wide. It felt liberating to lie on the earth again after spending so many winter months cooped up indoors. I drew several deep breaths into my belly and thought again about what Bonnie had said to me several days earlier: *You have so much to be grateful for.* Staring up at the white-gray clouds, I was instantly grateful for my eyesight. My mother was slowly losing hers to macular degeneration, and each time I visited her I could sense that her condition was getting worse. She often started out reading a newspaper or magazine upside down, and when she tried to look at a photograph through her magnifying glass she'd usually push it away with a deep sigh and say, "I just can't see it anymore. Tell me who's in it, will you?"

I was grateful that the EMDR treatments had taken the edge off of my visits with my parents. I no longer felt the intense anger and hurt that I used to feel: I was now more capable than ever of looking at them as two elderly people who had made some poor decisions when they were younger. There was no need to explain or defend or reinvent history. It was what it was. On that sunny spring day, I lay in the field and was grateful that they were still breathing and taking care of one another.

A half-hour later, I strolled toward the river that intersected our property and the state forest. I was a little wary of walking alone in the woods this time of year. The bears awoke from their winter hibernation in late March and early April, so it was always a good idea to scan the thawing mud for evidence of their scat or huge paw prints. A neighbor who knew every inch of the woods near our house had told me that bears ingest mud before they go to sleep for the winter.

"It plugs up their intestines," he explained. "It's the first thing they excrete when they wake up after a long winter and begin their search for food. You be sure to look for it. If you see some that looks fresh, just keep your eyes open and sing a little song while you're walking."

Keeping his advice in mind, I hiked through the woods singing and humming loudly while scanning the ground for any evidence of bear. The river was swollen with spring snowmelt and I sat in the middle of our homemade log bridge surveying the pine needles and twigs that swirled helplessly in the current. In the summer this small waterway dried up into a mere trickle but at this time of year it seemed more like the Colorado River; mini-rapids and frothing white caps raged beneath my feet. I wondered if the detritus would ever make it into the larger rivers and tributaries that eventually emptied into the Atlantic, or whether they'd wash up one day onto the shores of West Africa or southern Spain.

Walking back I tried to step as quietly as I imagined the moccasin-footed Native Americans did who used to inhabit these same paths four hundred years ago. For safety's sake I knew I should clap my hands and make loud noises to alert any bears that might be near, but the sound of the wind swaying through the pines had hypnotized me into silence. The remaining snow still crunched loudly beneath my boots but in the soft mud patches where new ferns were just springing up, I could take several steps without making a sound. As I crept slowly along the trail,

I suddenly heard a rustling noise. My heart stopped for a moment and a few seconds later I saw the flash of white tails and heard the pounding of hooves. Two does ran up and over a small rise not ten feet in front of me. I stood utterly still in mud up to my ankles and clenched my hands to my heart: I was thrilled at my startling encounter and most grateful that it had not been a bear.

The leaf canopy above my head was a luminescent green dome backlit by the intense afternoon sun. Staring up at it I remembered that a few years back I had been driving alone on one of the dirt roads when a majestic light-brown buck with a six-point set of antlers had come ambling out of the woods. I turned off the car engine and sat motionless behind the wheel watching him. The two of us stared at each other for what seemed like a very long time. Obviously skilled at avoiding hunters, he stood before me in proud and stately dignity. Neither one of us blinked until he finally turned his head away and walked slowly into the woods on the east side of the road.

When I lived in New York City, that kind of interaction used to happen all the time between strangers and me. Sitting side-by-side in close proximity to so many other people on a crowded subway, I often found myself reading someone else's book or newspaper right along with them. A slight nod of their head often let me know that it was okay with them. Or I might have dropped my purse on the sidewalk and before I knew it several considerate strangers were helping me corral my loose change before it rolled into the gutter. I still missed that kind of spontaneous human connection, but I was beginning to realize—perhaps because I was also longing to reconnect with my own lost animal self—that I was incredibly satisfied with and intrigued by the unpredictable interactions I had with nature.

Several years ago I had signed up for a workshop led by a shaman who had lived for ten years with Native Americans on reservations in New Mexico and Arizona. He had learned many spiritual and medicinal rituals from them, and this particular weekend we were exploring our animal totems. The Shaman began by asking us to close our eyes and imagine ourselves as an animal—any animal. I immediately envisioned myself as one of the lionesses Michael and I had spotted during a safari drive in the Serengeti years ago. My animal totem had big paws and a wide head and excellent vision.

"Familiarize yourself with your totem," he instructed us. "And then verbalize the language and sounds of the animal you have chosen."

We all looked at each other with trepidation. Did he really expect us to make animal noises in public? What was he thinking?

"Come on, folks," he encouraged us, "it's important to embody the animal totem, to own it in your soul."

Realizing that any resistance would be futile to the intention of the weekend, we all opened our mouths to roar, growl, bark, cluck, meow, hiss, coo, and neigh. We were a motley crew of dogs, cats, horses, tigers, prairie dogs, snakes, beetles, butterflies, and a dozen other creatures that roamed the planet. Our communal cacophony sounded like a five-o'clock traffic jam.

"In the course of our lives," he explained to us once we quieted down, "most people will discover that they have more than one totem. Different animals show up in our lives at different times and for different reasons. For example, the bear totem possesses the power of introspection, while the bobcat points to a solitary existence. Birds are survivalists. They will almost always choose flight over fight. Dogs teach people how to give and receive unconditionally."

He ran through a list of more than a dozen other totems, describing what they symbolized and how various cultures interpreted them. Lions were social creatures that supposedly taught humans lessons about group dynamics. Cows represented fertility and love, while bulls symbolized nourishment. Snakes were the universal sign of sexuality and life force, while the turtle was associated with longevity and connection to the earth. When he finished reviewing his lengthy totem list, he turned off all the lights and lit a single candle in the center of the circle we had formed. Then he asked us to close our eyes again but this time, instead of having us choose an animal, he wanted us to wait for an animal to choose us.

"Just sit quietly for a few minutes and wait and see what happens," he said in a hushed voice. "It is pointless to try to rush this process. Some of you may have to sit longer than others before the animal reveals itself. Just remember, this is also a lesson about allowing life to come to you rather than willing life to happen. Clues and messages arrive from the animal world all the time, but most often they are very subtle or disguised. We need to train ourselves to recognize them, and allow ourselves to learn from them."

I was quite happy to wait for a different animal to appear in my life. While roaring loudly like a lion in front of people I didn't know a few moments earlier, I had realized that I didn't really feel the need to be so aggressive anymore. I had been a lioness when I first moved to Manhattan—and for years before that. I had to be, in order to survive. The lioness had been my totem before I found pink, before my feminine side became just as powerful as my Yang side. Back then I was feisty, young, and strong and always ready for battle. But time had changed my outlook on life, and I guess it had affected my totem, too.

"What animal came to your mind, Miriam?" the Shaman asked when it was my turn to share with the group.

"This second time around I was a bit surprised that the lioness was nowhere in sight," I told them. "Instead I grew feathers and wings. I was a small bird perched high up in a tree taking in the big picture and not focusing on the details."

"That's excellent," he said. "Birds teach us awareness and adaptability, and they represent the air element. Songbirds teach us about proper breathing and the healing properties of sound."

When he asked us to emote the sound of our animal totems a second time, I was the only one in the group that exchanged my roar for a barely audible chirp. I had transformed into some kind of tiny being, like a sparrow or a finch.

As I made my way back to the house from the river, I wondered if I was still a bird or if I had morphed into something else entirely. Based on how I'd been feeling these last few months, I thought that maybe I was some kind of swamp animal, perhaps a lizard or a bullfrog. I had abruptly cut the chord with my warm-blooded animal-self months ago when I realized that I would never experience the bittersweet ritual of pregnancy and labor. Having served as a birthing coach twice in my life, I had witnessed firsthand the ways in which the women I attended shifted from human to animal as their labors progressed. Those remarkable experiences had left me marveling about the mysteries of evolution and the transmutation of the human form and soul. After careful consideration, I decided that I was still a bird but no longer a small one. I had graduated into a larger wingspan of four to five feet and I flew swiftly and confidently through the shadow sky; I was an owl—the symbol of the feminine, the moon, and the night.

Owl Medicine was traditionally used to guide people through the darkest night and lead them back to their proper path. The Owl was crucial for clearing out that which was no longer needed, and for helping people to recognize that what may have seemed like the death of one dream was actually the birth of something unexpected and new. That interpretation of the owl totem made total sense to me: in a few short months a son or daughter would arrive in our lives, and I would become a wise and compassionate mother. I was humbled and most grateful for that.

❖

With a cup of ginger tea in my hand, I sat in the rocking chair on the porch and watched the clouds roll in. The weather forecast had predicted thunderstorms, and I could see a dark line forming on the horizon. Within an hour, fat drops of rain were pelting against the windows, and thunder rumbled across the valley. Possessed by spring fever and the need to feel fresh water on my skin, I stripped off all my clothes and stood naked in the rain. Steam rose off my skin like smoke, and when the light show began I wrapped myself in a towel and sat back in the rocking chair to watch.

Long, crooked bolts of lightning flashed in the sky followed by the deafening sound of thunderclaps so loud they shook the rafters of our house. It was the second most ferocious storm I had ever encountered, the first being a hurricane that hit unexpectedly when I was camping with my family on the Delaware shore as a kid. I had spent a terrified night in the car while my parents tried to keep the tent from blowing away. As frightening as that experience was, it had taught me to appreciate the beauty and power of storms. During the blizzard of 1978—an infamous Nor'easter that dumped close to six feet of snow on the East Coast—Bonnie and I had driven an hour through blinding conditions and treacherous roads to watch huge waves crash onto the beaches north of Gloucester. It was a storm of Biblical proportions; the winds blew a steady eighty-nine miles per hour with gusts up to 111. Severe coastal flooding caused hundreds of homes to wash away into oblivion. It was thrilling to witness.

Michael shared my passion for storms, and we sometimes planned our weekends around them. We loved riding the ferry during high seas and always seemed to stake out the best spot on the bow. Waves often crashed fifteen feet up from the waterline, drenching us with salt and spray and leaving us laughing and awestruck by the supremacy of the sea. When he was running the hotel during the summer months at Cape Cod, he was always eager to host Hurricane Parties. He and his crew would board up the windows of the restaurant with plywood, light kerosene lanterns, and make Hot Toddies. Someone inevitably strummed a guitar or a banjo, and when the winds picked up and the rain poured down, we'd all run across the street to the beach in our bathing suits and dive into the pounding surf.

"Hold onto my hand tight," Michael would scream to me over the roar of the wind and waves that whipped at our wet hair and bodies. "Don't let go of my hand. There's big undertow and storm surge here. Ready? Here we go." And with big smiles on our faces we'd run as fast as we could and plunge head first inside the curl of a wave before its frothy crest crashed over our heads.

Watching the storm from the safety of the porch at our house, I humbly acknowledged that these last six years had been the most threatening storms Michael and I had ever weathered. We knew so many couples who had been ripped apart by failed treatments and other life crises. It was so easy and sometimes incredibly tempting to just let go and see where life would take you, like the pine needles floating downstream in the river. In those fleeting moments when I imagined Michael and me living separate lives again, I drifted back to Africa and worked at an orphanage or imagined myself speaking fluent Italian and riding my Vespa past the Coliseum in Rome. Michael had his share of daydreams that didn't include me, either. A couple of months earlier, he had announced that he was going to captain a retired marine research vessel and conduct experiments to figure out how to harness the power of the ocean into renewable energy.

What amazed me most when I thought back over the events of the last seventy-two months was the fact that we never did let go of each other's hands, and I am grateful for that. Even during the most trying and doubtful times of our marriage, we *always* made sure that at least our little fingers or big toes were touching. One or both of us always took care to ensure that the circle would not be broken. When the fog was so thick we could not possibly rely on our senses to confirm our existence, we made sure that we went to bed every night feeling loved and connected. Now that that phase of our life was finally fading, we were starting to regain our energy. We were looking toward the future, planning new adventures and staying focused on the notion that we would become parents when the Abstract Love Child of Our Dreams was ready to manifest. Our hearts and arms were wide open for that child to drop out of the sky.

As the lightning struck and the thunder boomed across the sky, I smiled as I thought about the magnificent resilience of the human spirit to rise up time and time again in the face of adversity and hardship. Knowing firsthand about that was as inspiring as the electric storm dancing across the sky in front of me: Mother Nature once again reigned victorious.

STORKS

By early June, Michael and I were starting to feel a bit like our old, happy selves. When the invitation to attend my friend's daughter's wedding in North Africa arrived, we both smiled.

"We're going—right?" Michael asked when I showed him the invitation.

"Of course," I replied. "I already spoke to the agency and Linda said it is unlikely that anything will happen anytime soon. They said we should book the tickets."

Freddy's daughter Meredith had graduated from Georgetown University with a degree in French and had been expanding her language repertoire—which also included Russian, Italian, and Spanish—by learning Arabic. She had met the groom-to-be, Abdel, while teaching English in Rabat, Morocco, and bartending on the weekends in the trendy tourist city of Marrakesh. The traditional Islamic-Western wedding ceremony was to be held in an ornate mosaic castle in the heart of the nation's capital on July fourteenth. Festivities would commence with a Henna Party at the groom's mother's house and conclude at four a.m. the following day.

The week before we left, our dear friend Melissa and her daughter, Natasha, came for a whirlwind visit from Atlanta. One afternoon Tashi begged us to go to the M.S.P.C.A. Dog Rescue so she could visit with the canines waiting for families to adopt them.

"I know we have Martin King at home, Mom, but maybe we should get another dog, you know, to keep him company."

Melissa rolled her eyes, thinking of their 100-pound Burmese Mountain Dog, a majestic beast with paws the size of baseball mitts, who spent most of his days lying on the cool tile floor of their air-conditioned house.

"Don't get your hopes up too high, Tashi," Melissa advised as she covered her nose with a handkerchief to ward off the serious stench of wet dog that enveloped us as soon as we walked through the shelter door. As usual, there were several sweet-looking pit bulls whose reputation for violence—whether earned or not—would likely lead to their demise. Accompanying them was an old, squat dog with dappled fur and cataracts who pressed his black nose to the glass and stared at us with sad, forlorn eyes. His family had moved away and left him behind in their old apartment.

"Adopt me, please," he seemed to say. "Don't leave me here alone."

As we exited to the parking lot gulping big breaths of fresh air, my cell phone rang. It was Linda.

"Hi," I said tentatively, wondering why she was calling.

"Is Michael with you?"

"Yes."

"Well, that's good, because I have good news for you."

My heart stopped.

"You do?" we asked in unison, looking at each other with wide eyes.

"A birth mother has selected you to become parents."

"The magic words," I thought to myself, squeezing Michael's hand.

"This is for real?" he asked Linda.

"Very real," she said. "She and her family know that you are leaving for Morocco on Friday so they all want to meet you tomorrow at two p.m. in our office. Can you make it?"

"We'll be there," Michael said. "But maybe we should just cancel the trip? We don't have to go."

"No, no. Don't cancel," Linda said. "You never know how these things will work out. I'd hate for you to cancel the trip and then have the adoption fall through. You both need to exercise what we like to call Cautious Optimism."

"Right," we said. "Cautious Optimism. See you tomorrow."

Twenty-four hours later we met M., the young woman who had read through our adoption photo album and decided that we should raise her son. She was a beautiful, healthy, smiling twenty-one-year-old with long, straight black hair and bright, twinkling eyes. Despite all the angst we assumed she was experiencing, she appeared to be happy and confident. She was due to deliver a week after we returned from our trip. I sat directly across from her during the meeting, my eyes riveted on the bulge of her belly where her baby—my potential son—now lived.

I do believe that striking a balance of Cautious Optimism is one of the most difficult emotional states for anyone to master. Doctors advise cancer patients to remain "cautiously optimistic" about chemotherapy treatments arresting their disease. And diplomats negotiating peace agreements between warring parties often announce during press conferences that they are "cautiously optimistic" about reaching a cease-fire agreement. Michael and I weren't quite sure how we were supposed to carve out that emotional space within ourselves. Each moment we had to force ourselves to stay anchored in the here and now, and to resist our minds' temptations to map out the baby's entire future.

"M. has prepared a set of questions she'd like to ask you," her social worker explained. I nodded to M. with a humble smile, fighting off my own urge to ask her a million questions. I wanted to know more about her, so that when her son grew up and asked about his birth mother I would be able to tell him what her favorite color and flower were, what kind of music she liked, and what kind of books she read. Did she love the ocean or the mountains or big cities? Was her favorite meal spaghetti and meatballs or baked scallops? I knew nothing about this pregnant stranger, and yet, if we did become parents to her son, we would be linked to her for the rest of our lives.

"What would you do if when the baby grew up he told you he didn't want to go to college?" M. asked Michael.

"I'd help him figure out other avenues of learning," he responded. "I'd help him embrace his talents and earn a living doing something that he loved to do."

"Okay," she said, smiling at him. "I asked that question because I'm not sure what I want to do with my life. Sometimes it's hard to figure that out."

Then, turning to me, she asked: "If you had the choice between watching TV with the baby or reading him books, what would you choose?"

"I'm not a big fan of television," I told her. "Most likely I will read him book after book after book." She smiled back at me for that answer, too, her eyes sparkling. I wondered how she felt just then. I assumed she trusted us. She had to—otherwise I'm not sure she could let go. I wanted her to know that we were loyal to her cause, like the Knights of the Round Table were loyal to Arthur and Camelot. On blind faith, M. was entrusting us to love and cherish her son, and we both felt that raising him was a sacred responsibility. Maybe we had walked our not so easy path—with fertility and with each other—in order to finally meet M. and her son. If things went as planned, we would be a "family" in the most universal meaning of the word.

◆

Still thinking we were insane for leaving the country, we flew to Morocco the next day, arriving just in time to have drinks with other members of the wedding party who were staying at the same hotel. There were three attractive, long-legged young women—Tatia, Nino, and Nino (yes—believe it or not both women were named Nino)— from the country of Georgia, dressed in mini-skirts and high heels, who seemed not to notice the more conservative dress code of the Muslim women swarming around them in headscarves and robes. Then there were Anna and Camilla, Freddy's beautiful cousins from Rome; Meredith's mother, Sandy, and her stepfather, Al; and Freddy and his lovely wife, P.J. For the next five days, we moved as one organism through the old and new neighborhoods of the city, visiting ancient ruins and bartering with merchants in the markets.

My favorite site was the ruins of Chellah, a mix of crumbling Roman and Arabic stone structures perched on a hill looking out onto the Atlantic Coast. We strolled through the gardens, past exotic flowers like bird of paradise and hibiscus, and watched packs of feral cats play with ripe oranges that had fallen from the trees. At one point the garden footpath gave way to open space, and that was when we saw them: hundreds of white storks nesting in the treetops that lined the edge of the castle's perimeter. They clacked their beaks like chopsticks in a wild symphony of sound, and, when they spread their broad wings to fly, their outermost feathers looked like they had been dipped in black ink.

"I know we're not supposed to believe in omens anymore," I said to Michael, as we stood side by side looking at the sea of white birds. "But don't you think this is a good sign?"

"No," he said quickly, with obvious irritation in his voice. "They're just birds, remember? They aren't magical apparitions telling us that we'll become parents when we go home. They are what they are: a bunch of big white birds sitting in big stick nests and crapping all over the sidewalk."

"But you always said, 'If only a stork would deliver a baby onto our pillow you would gladly call it your own and be its father.' That time may really be now."

"Please don't start clinging to superstitions and animal totems again," said my formerly mystical husband before walking away to have his photo taken with Tatia, who looked like a *Vogue* model. "You know how dangerous that can be." He was right to exercise Cautious Optimism. He was protecting himself. As I looked around at the remnants of 2,000-year-old ruins that used to house the scholars of the royal family, I decided that the presence of the storks *was* a favorable omen; if I was wrong, then the crushing blow would be mine to bear alone.

Later that afternoon, we went to Abdel's mother's home for the customary pre-nuptial Henna Party. It was an honor to be invited into Naima's apartment, decorated with mosaic tiles and ornate carved plaster ceilings. Banks of red and gold couches laden with embroidered pillows adorned the edges of the living room, leaving a large open space in the middle for dancing and mingling. Several of Abdel's relatives were already there when we arrived, mostly older women wearing head-scarves and black robes, but other women were dressed in colorful satin gowns with plunging necklines and side slits that allowed easy movement for dancing. That day I learned that, robed or not, these women were extremely sensual dancers, swaying their hips and shimmying their torsos in ways that were much more seductive than your typical rock 'n' roll dance in the States.

The wedding itself began at nine p.m. the following day, in a castle nestled deep inside the city. We were all dumbstruck by the beauty of the architecture, and the way the candles lit in every room illuminated the intricate mosaic patterns. The acoustics from the two bands, one playing lively African-Moroccan dance music and the other more staid American jazz, echoed throughout the building as though it were a cave. The singers' voices and the eerie notes of the electric violin ascended upwards and then bounced back down to the floor. Men costumed in dramatic red capes and gold fez hats carried the bride and groom around the courtyard on big silver platters while trumpeters heralded their arrival on six-foot-long brass horns. Meredith looked like a princess, with her rhinestone tiaras and three different costume changes: a customary white Moroccan dress covered by a sheer tunic embroidered with gold flowers, a traditional long-sleeved crimson-and-gold satin kaftan, and finally a strapless white satin gown, reminiscent of what Grace Kelly wore in the film *To Catch a Thief*. All through the night, Michael and I kept smiling at each other, knowing that we were witnessing twenty-first-century rituals that resembled something right out of *The Arabian Nights*. We also knew that, if the adoption moved forward as we hoped it would, we would one day be able to tell our little boy about the night we attended a Moroccan wedding.

❖

Once back in the States, we checked in with the agency to make sure we hadn't been dreaming about M. choosing us to be parents to her child.

"She still thinks you two are great," Linda told us in a calm voice. "Everything is in order. All we have to do is wait for the baby to be born."

Michael and I looked at each other with alarm, realizing that we had a million things to do in *four* days. We had only recently painted the nursery, which was completely empty except for a hammer and screwdriver that sat on one of the windowsills. That week we made ten trips to Target and Babies "R" Us, walking up and down each aisle with glazed eyes and confused minds. Our pending parenthood was as foreign to us as Morocco had been, but we needed to plunge into it and learn its preparatory nuances immediately. We loaded our carts with diapers, bottles, nipples, strollers, changing tables, burp clothes, thermometers, socks, blankets, stuffed animals, and a few hundred other items we didn't know what to do with. Then we remembered we needed to choose a name for the baby.

"Any ideas?" I asked Michael.

"Jebediah," he said with a nod of his head.

"Jebediah?" I said, my mouth hanging open in horror. "You want to call my son Jebediah?"

"That's right, little lady," he replied, feigning a baritone fire-and-brimstone preacher voice. "We're going to name him Jebediah and he will walk upon this earth for many years to come."

"I don't think so," I told him. "It sounds so over-the-top Old Testament."

After drinking two bottles of wine during a delicious Italian dinner, we finally reached an agreement. With big smiles on our faces and tears in our eyes, we decided that if this little boy ever did find us we would name him Samuel Victor Shashoua.

"I like it," Michael said as the last drop of wine trickled from his glass onto his lip. "It's a dignified, solid name." Now, as Linda had said days earlier, we just had to wait for Sam to be born.

❖

The phone finally did ring. It was Linda.

"M. is in labor, and she's in the hospital."

"Oh my God," I said. "It's really happening, then?"

"Yes, it's really happening," she replied.

"How can you be so calm?"

"That's my job—remember? I'll call you the minute I hear anything."

"Okay," I said, hanging up the phone.

"What? What? What's going on?" Michael asked.

"M. is in labor," I told him. "Sam may be born today or tomorrow, which means we'll bring him home Thursday or Friday."

We both stared at each other, unable to speak, realizing that the end of our seven-year search for our Holy Grail was imminent.

"Are we dreaming?" Michael asked in a quiet voice.

"I think it's real," I said, squeezing his hand.

Later that evening Linda called to tell us that Samuel had been born via C-section at six p.m., weighing in at a whopping nine pounds six ounces.

"He's a big, healthy baby," she told us. "M. is resting comfortably and recovering from surgery. It looks like you'll be able to bring him home on Friday."

❖

The moment I laid eyes on Sammy, a force of maternal instinct that I had never felt before welled up inside of me like a great tsunami.

"That's my baby," I thought to myself possessively, drinking in the tiny image of him sitting in bed next to his birthmother. He felt so familiar to me, as though I had met him before, or dreamed about him a thousand times. Though I did not suffer through the pains of labor as M. had, I did believe that somehow this small being also sprang forth from the spiritual cocoon spun from my long-held prayers. I had to fight off my surprisingly intense Mama Bear instincts to immediately grab him, and when M. finally asked if we wanted to hold him, I let Michael cradle Sammy first. I held my breath, afraid that the whole scene might evaporate before my eyes. When it was finally my turn, my chest trembled as I looked down into his perfectly formed face. I still couldn't quite comprehend that he was "my son" and that I was now "his mother." In an *instant*, we had all assumed new identities that would bind us to one another for life.

I was at once humbled and grateful sitting next to M., whose eyes were red and puffy from crying. She loved Sammy as much as we did. There was no question about that. I looked at her then and wondered if she could possibly comprehend the level of gratitude that her decision had brought to my heart. Her courage to place him in our solid arms was one of the bravest acts I had ever witnessed.

That night I gave Sammy his five a.m. bottle. It was just the two of us awake in the early morning calm. I chuckled to myself at the irony of finally becoming a mother at the ripe old age of forty-six. Michael and I had spent seven frustrating years trying to conceive naturally and artificially, but only seven months in the adoption process before we became parents. When all was said and done, the biggest lesson I had learned was that of giving up on the idea that you can control anything in this world. It's a hard thing to do, but if you can do that, then you can actually accept where you are and be at peace with it. Most of the time, whether we know it or not, we are in a beautiful, perfect place. For me right now, it is right here, listening to the sound of my son cooing softly as the sun rises.

AFTERWORD

We were like all new parents: Sammy's arrival brought joy, chaos, and exhaustion into our lives. Engulfed by diapers, formula, and formidable loads of laundry, I placed this manuscript on a shelf and tried really hard to forget about it. I was a mother. Like so many women who have lived through failed treatments, I didn't want to think about the hardships of the last seven years. I was cradling my tiny son and he was reaching for my mouth with his little fingers, locking his eyes onto mine! I was smitten, living fulltime in Baby Land. I refused to leave the farm. Crickets hummed and bees buzzed and all was perfect, as it should be.

And then the bubble burst. Alongside my overwhelming feelings of gratitude and wonder toward his birthmother and the miracle of this new life, I reluctantly admitted that I was still grieving over what hadn't happened through fertility treatments. I would steal glances at Sammy and feel ashamed that I was still carrying that load. I felt as if I were betraying him, and Michael, and the sweetness of our new family dynamic. I tried to brush away the feelings, but they kept creeping back in, tucking themselves right alongside my new-mother emotions, where they coexisted for a while.

When I finally ventured out of Baby Land into the real world again, I felt blinded by the light and noise of everyday life. With the privilege of motherhood I had intentionally buried my head in the sand and taken a sabbatical from news of bloody wars and economic down-turns. Now that I was coming out of hiding, I felt extremely vulnerable. Knowing that I needed help to move on, I sought out a business coach and a counselor. I was disheartened when session after session dredged up the guilt and shame and remorse I still felt. I needed to forgive myself for missing the opportunity to birth a child. Thanks to more somatic treatments like EMDR and Thought Field Therapy, some of my physiological triggers did begin to dissipate, but others remained, and as I wrestled with my lingering demons, I sensed that I was not alone.

The study by Allyson Bradow that I referenced earlier (also see *Resources*) is the only study I have come across linking post-traumatic stress disorder (PTSD) to women whose fertility treatments failed them. While other psychological literature acknowledges the strain and grief involved during treatments—many even compare them to cancer treatments—none that I know is so bold. For many of these women, whose infertility was linked to age not genetics, myself included, the promise of reproductive technologies figured prominently from an early age in the way we mapped out the trajectory of our lives. We would spend so many years in college, so many years in graduate school; hopefully we would find a mate early on, but, even if we didn't, we could build our professional standing and income knowing that we could rely on science to help us become mothers in our late thirties or early forties. This pattern of thinking was embedded in our culture: endorsed by the medical community and reinforced by the media. To learn later, after painful personal experience, that the vast majority of reproductive technologies do not, in fact, result in live births is a double tragedy. Not only are we coping with the loss of a deep primal desire to birth offspring, we must also come to terms with the fact that we built our entire "women-can-finally-have-it-all" adult life on an illusion.

The current clinical definition of PTSD applies to people who have experienced or witnessed a life-threatening event or an event that could cause serious injury, but Bradow suggests that the definition be expanded to include expectations of life. "Having children, expanding your family, and carrying on your genetic code—that's an instinctual drive that we have as human beings. When that is being threatened, it's not necessarily your life being threatened, but your expectation of what your life can be or should be like."

As one participant in the study wrote:

> There is an empty, useless, and sad feeling in my heart nearly every day. Some days I feel stronger and normal, but little everyday things… walking in a store and passing the baby section or a pregnant woman, a diaper commercial, etc., will set me off and I'll feel broken all over again. This has been going on for over fifteen years with me.

Bradow's study confirmed for me that, just because the doctor appointments, the injections, the egg transfers, and the dashed hopes are over, it does not mean that the trauma is over. The sense of violation that many women say they still feel years later, coupled with the deep, deep sadness of not having borne a child, lingers in our lives like a persistent mosquito buzzing in a dark room. Even when you don't hear it you know it is there, waiting to sting you, and it does.

❖

With Sammy stowed safely in his baby carrier, I would stand in line at the grocery store and try to shield myself from the never-ending onslaught of misleading and sensationalized media headlines that had initially pulled me into treatments. Still missing from most mainstream news coverage were thoughtful analyses of the complex ramifications these unprecedented technologies were wreaking in the lives of millions of families around the globe, not to mention modern society at large. Each time a headline caught my eye I would turn away from it with a fierce intention to disconnect and disassociate, until one day a friend told me about a woman she knew who had spent ten years in treatments and finally did birth a daughter.

This woman had recently decided to venture back to the clinic to try to conceive a second child. The three fertilized embryos eventually implanted in her womb all clung to her for dear life, but then she was advised by her doctors that, if they did not terminate two of them, they could risk losing them all. My heart went out to this woman, whom I imagined sitting on the edge of her bed staring at the floor and weeping. "How can it be," she might whisper to herself as she held her belly, "that I must now choose which embryo will blossom into new life and which ones will never see the light of day?"

That particular story was the one that motivated me to finish this book. By disclosing my personal experience, I'm hoping that others will begin to speak out and share theirs, whether treatments were successful or not. For those still recovering, I invite you to cast off your silence and contribute to expanding an open and honest consumer-driven discussion about these life-altering technologies. Men and women contemplating fertility treatments need to hear your perspective, as do those who are working with clinics to improve the way they interact with and support patients, donors, and surrogates. By sharing your experiences with friends, family, and the media, you will help create a more balanced perspective and understanding of reproductive medicine and the extreme challenges facing those who opt for treatments. (If you would like to share information about your experience with the voluntary registry at Dartmouth Hitchcock Medical Center, please visit www.ifrr-registry.org)

Couples who have difficulty conceiving and turn to reproductive technology for help deserve access to accurate and easy-to-decipher data about clinic failure and success rates. This data needs to be calculated by all clinics through uniform methods and reported to the CDC through standardized mechanisms. Those entering into treatments also need exposure to the most up-to-date studies addressing potential health risks, and to current legal, bioethical, philosophical, and spiritual debates concerning the reach and ramifications of these new discoveries. That said, more money must be invested in research to assess the short- and long-term health vulnerabilities facing women undergoing treatments––and the children born from them. It is also time to establish an external oversight authority focused on consumer protections that will objectively scrutinize new technologies, evaluate current practices, and make enforceable health and safety recommendations.

Over the last thirty-five years the powerful combination of reproductive medicines' marketing strategies and the mainstream media's tendency to overestimate the potential of new technologies has led to a global epidemic of misinformation about the age when women's fertility naturally declines and about the power of modern medicine to reverse it. The studies from four countries that I cited earlier in the book confirm this. What's needed now is a revamping of the way we educate young adults—and the general population—about the lifespan of their reproductive capacities, and about infertility in general. If we want, in particular, to prevent age-related involuntary childlessness in the future, we must equip young people the world over with accurate information about their fertility so they can plan accordingly for their journey toward parenthood—if they so choose. One of the best ways to accomplish this is to reeducate doctors who interact annually with patients of reproductive age about women and men's fertility peaks and declines. Obstetricians and gynecologists, in particular, need to be encouraged to provide women with the facts about their biology, and to supply them with accurate information about the failure and success rates of reproductive technology.

Finally, in more recent years, the cultural promotion of reproductive medicine as the primary solution to infertility has often overshadowed the ancient and established role that adoption has always played in helping couples build their families. The spiritual value and emotional rewards of adoption as a primary alternative to childlessness need to continue to remain essential parts of the conversation for those trying to determine what path to parenthood is best for them. Speaking from our own experience, Michael and I could not imagine a deeper, more sacred and fulfilling bond than the one we have with our beautiful son.

ACKNOWLEDGEMENTS

There are many people who have lent me support, suggestions, and a shoulder to lean on during the long and often grueling process of writing this book.

First and foremost I would like to thank my husband, Michael Shashoua, for being open to the idea of sharing our deeply personal growing pains with the world. Our journey together continues to unfold in unpredictable ways that test and teach us surprising lessons about love and the notion of staying connected "through thick and thin." A big, big thanks, as well, to my beautiful little boy, Sammy, who makes my heart whole and whose love and laughter enrich my life every day.

My dear friend Meryl Levin carved out huge chunks of time in her hectic new-mother schedule and beyond to converse with me night and day about the mysteries of the drive to procreate. Shelley Eriksen and Jackson and Judah Katz arrived for sabbatical twice in western Massachusetts when I most needed their friendship, thoughtfulness, and editorial suggestions. My wise friend Leigh Bailey and her unflappable husband, Joel Spiro, spent hundreds of hours over the course of several years helping me wade through the sociological and bioethical minefields of my own, and society's, use of reproductive technologies. My friend and colleague Micol Zarb provided feedback on early drafts of the book, as did Will Kanteres and Matthew Carnicelli, whose unwavering support and editorial wisdom inspired me to soothe the rawness in my heart and create closure. Sally Whelan served as a sounding board and offered suggestions for an almost-finished manuscript; Monique Hillen showered me with empathy, insight, and intuition; and Allyson Bradow validated my post-ART existence by offering evidence about the relationship between failed fertility treatments and severe trauma. Sut Jhally, founder and executive director of the Media Education Foundation and professor of communications at the University of Massachusetts-Amherst, made important introductions and connections on my behalf.

I am grateful to my publisher, Michel Moushabeck, and his team at Interlink Publishing, who asked tough questions and helped me bring this book into the world where it can hopefully help expand the much needed public discourse about reproductive technologies' growing influence in our world. I would like to acknowledge the support of my parents, Nathan and Jacquelyn Zoll; my sister, Rachel; and my brother, Daniel, who encouraged me to write about many of the challenges we faced together as a family. The care and concern of my gregarious in-laws—Tribe Shashoua—helped sustain me during difficult times and beyond. Thanks also to my high school English teacher, Sandra Smeltzer, who taught me how to honor my life experiences and write from the heart. A big thanks to my dedicated yoga students in Ashfield, Massachusetts, for showing up for classes even when I thought I couldn't, and to the Forbes Library and the libraries at Smith College in Northampton, MA where I camped out for days at a time to write.

READING GROUP QUESTIONS AND
TOPICS FOR DISCUSSION

1. Before reading *Cracked Open*, what were your general impressions about fertility treatments and the people who used them? Do any particular headlines from media coverage come to mind?

2. What did you think about the doctors' suggestion that women should be finished with childbearing by age 35? Do you know women like Miriam who felt the need to postpone motherhood? Were their experiences similar to the author's?

3. What did you think when Miriam and Michael decided to begin using IVF? Would you ever consider using these treatments for yourself, or recommend them to someone you know? Why or why not?

4. Miriam references the generational differences between herself and her mother many times in the book. What are these differences and how do they apply to your own experience?

5. What was the most interesting aspect of Miriam and Michael's relationship? What did you find most amusing about their adventure living in the country?

6. What was your reaction to Miriam and Michael's miscarriage?

7. In the chapter *Finding Pink*, Miriam acknowledges that she spent many years turning away from her feminine side because she equated

it with women's lack of power in the world. What do you think about some of the choices she made? Have you made similar choices? What were they?

8. The author discusses her discomfort about being in the position to select traits for her offspring. What are your feelings about egg donation? Sperm donation? Do you think it is important to account for the numbers of children being born through donor technology? To track their health and development? Why or why not?

9. What was your reaction when you learned that both egg donors were infertile?

10. The author relates her ambivalence about monitoring the fertility industry because she fears it might trespass on women's reproductive rights. At the same time, she believes that women undergoing treatments—and their potential offspring—need more protections. How do you feel about this? What are your major concerns?

11. Can you relate to the depression the author experienced? What events in your life have triggered similar experiences for you? How did you cope during difficult times?

12. What did you learn about adoption as a result of reading *Cracked Open*? Do you have any personal experiences with children who are adopted?

RESOURCES AND REFERENCES

Counseling Services

EMDR International Association (Eye Movement Desensitization and Reprocessing)
5806 Mesa Drive, Suite 360
Austin, TX 78731
www.emdria.org
Phone: (512) 451-5200
Toll-free: (866)451-5200
Fax: (512) 451-5256
E-mail: info@emdria.org

The Trauma Center at Justice Resource Center
1269 Beacon Street
Brookline, MA 02446
Phone: (617) 232-1303
www.traumacenter.org

American Association of Sexuality Educators, Counselors and Therapists (AASECT)
1444 I Street NW, Suite 700
Washington, DC 20005
Phone: (202) 449-1099 Fax: (202) 216-9646
http://www.aasect.org

Films

Eggsploitation
The Center for Bioethics and Culture Network
130 Market Place, #146
San Ramon, CA 94583
E-mail: cbcinfo@cbc-network.org

Made in India (international surrogacy, reproductive tourism)
E-mail: info@madeinindiamovie.com

Organizations

United States
Our Bodies, Ourselves
5 Upland Road, #3
Cambridge, MA 02140
Phone: (617) 245-0200
www.ourbodiesourselves.org

Infertility Family Research Registry Department of Ob/Gyn
Dartmouth-Hitchcock Medical Center
One Medical Center Drive
Lebanon, NH 03756
Phone: (603) 653-9900
www.ifrr-registry.org

The Center for Genetics in Society
1936 University Ave, Suite 350,
Berkeley, CA 94704
Phone: (510) 625-0819
Fax: (510) 665-8760
E-mail: info@geneticsandsociety.org
www.genetics-and-society.org

Pro Choice Alliance for Responsible Research (PCARR)
Public Health Institute
1825 Bell Street, Suite 203
Sacramento, CA 95825
E-mail: info@prochoicealliance.org
www.prochoicealliance.org

Council for Responsible Genetics
30 Broad Street, 30th Fl.
New York, NY 10004
Phone: (212) 361-6360
www.councilforresponsiblegenetics.org

The UCLA Institute for Society and Genetics
Box 957221
1323 Rolfe Hall
Los Angeles, CA 90095-7221
Campus mailcode: 722102
Phone: (310) 267-4990
Fax: (310) 206-1880
E-mail: socgen@socgen.ucla.edu

The Donor Sibling Registry
PO Box 1571
Nederland, CO 80466
www.donorsiblingregistry.com
Phone: (303) 280-5267

India (reproductive tourism)
SAMA–Resource Group for Women and Health
2nd Floor, B 45, Shivalik Main, Malviya Nagar
New Delhi, India 110017
Phone: +9111 65637632, 26692730
E-mail: sama.womenshealth@gmail.com
sama.genderhealth@gmail.com

Nepal (reproductive tourism)
WOREC (Women's Rights in Nepal)
P. O. Box 13233
Balkumari, Lalitpur
Phone: +977-1-5006373, 5006374
E-mail: ics@worecnepal.org

Israel
Women and Their Bodies
E-mail: info@wtb.co.il

Japan
Miho Ogino, Shokado Women's Bookstore
E-mail: mihogino@polka.plala.or.jp
www.ourbodiesourselves.org/programs/network/foreign/japan.asp

Chile and Puerto Rico
Nirvana Gonzalez Rosa
E-mail: nirvanag@caribe.net

References

Bradow, Allyson. "Primary and Secondary Infertility and Post Traumatic Stress Disorder: Experiential Differences Between Type of Infertility and Symptom Characteristics." Ph. D diss., the School of Psychology, Spalding University, 2010.

Bretherick, Karla. "Fertility and Aging: Do Reproductive-Aged Canadian Women Know What They Need to Know?" *Fertility and Sterility*, Volume 93, Issue 7 (May 2010): 2162-68.

Centers for Disease Control www.cdc.gov/art

Cohen, Margot. "A Search for Surrogates Leads to India." *Wall Street Journal*, October 2009.

"Epidemic of Older Mothers." *British Medical Journal*, Vol. 331 (November 2005): 588-9.

European Society for Human Reproduction and Embryology www.eshre.eu/

"Fertility Treatment Bans in Europe Raise Controversy, Questions." *CBS News*, April 13, 2012.

Hashiloni-Dolev, Y. "The Fertility Myth: Israeli Students' Knowledge Regarding Age-Related Fertility Decline and Late Pregnancies in an Era of Assisted Reproduction Technology." *Human Reproduction* (September 2011): 3045-53. E-publication.

Indian Council of Medical Research, http://www.icmr.nic.in/
Jain, Tarun. "Significant disparities exist among patients seeking access to infertility treatment in a state with mandated insurance coverage." *Fertility and Sterility*, July 2005.

Lampic, C., et al. "Fertility Awareness, Intentions Concerning Childbearing, and Attitudes Towards Parenthood Among Female and Male Academics (Sweden)." *Human Reproduction*, Vol. 21, No. 2 (November 17, 2005): 558-64.
Maranto, Gina, "The Abiding 'Fertility Myth." *Biopolitical Times*, November 9, 2011, www.biopoliticaltimes.org/article.php?id=5929

Millheiser, Leah, et al. "Is Infertility a Risk Factor for Female Sexual Dysfunction? A Case-Control Study." *Fertility and Sterility*, Vol. 94, No. 6 (November 2010): 2022-25.

Orenstein, Peggy, "Your Gamete, Myself," *New York Times Magazine*, July 2007, http://www.nytimes.com/2007/07/15/magazine/15eggt.html?r=2&oref=slogin&

Peterson, Brennan D., Matthew Pirritano, Laura Tucker, and Claudia Lampic. "Fertility Awareness and Parenting Attitudes Among American Male and Female Undergraduate University Students." *Human Reproduction*, Vol. 27, No. 5 (March 8, 2012): 1375-82.

Salmon, Andrew, "Hwang Woo-suk: Rise and Fall of Korea's Most Famed Scientist," *Korea Times*, April 4, 2012, http://www.koreatimes.co.kr/www/news/nation/2012/10/363_108769.html

Schubert, Charlotte, "Egg Freezing Enters Clinical Mainstream,"*Nature* Magazine, October 23, 2012, http://www.scientificamerican.com/article.cfm?id=egg-freezing-enters-clinical-mainstream.

NOTES

[1] Neergaard, Lauran. "Doctors Aim to Save Fertility of Kids with Cancer." *Associated Press*, March 10.

[2] RESOLVE, http://www.resolve.org/about/fast-facts-about-fertility.html

[3] Centers for Disease Control, http://www.cdc.gov/nchs/fastats/fertile.htm, data from National Survey of Family Growth (2006-2010).

[4] *Assisted Reproductive Technology (ART)*, Ctr. Disease Control (last updated Aug.1, 2012).

[5] Kornblum, Janet. "More Women 40-44 Remaining Childless." *USA Today*, August 19, 2008.

[6] Peterson, Brennan D., Matthew Pirritano, Laura Tucker, and Claudia Lampic. "Fertility Awareness and Parenting Attitudes Among American Male and Female Undergraduate University Students." *Human Reproduction*, Vol. 27, No.5 (March 8, 2012): 1375-82.

[7] http://www.fertilitycommunity.com/fertility/asrms-infertility-preventioncampaign.html

[8] http://www.biopoliticaltimes.org/article.php?id=4496